Mystical Aromatherapy

The Divine Gift of Fragrance

BY: AVRAHAM SAND

LOTUS PRESS
P.O. Box 325
Twin Lakes, WI 53181 USA

Author: Avraham Sand
www.AvAroma.com

First Edition 2012

Printed in the United States of America

ISBN: 978-0-9406-7694-7

Library of Congress Number: 2011929094

LOTUS PRESS

Published by:
Lotus Press, P.O. Box 325, Twin Lakes, WI 53181 USA
web: www.lotuspress.com
Email: lotuspress@lotuspress.com
800.824.6396

Table of Contents

Introduction

I am a professional Aromatherapist, as well as a *Cohen* – a direct descendant of Aaron, the original High Priest, whose ceremonial responsibilities included burning the Temple Incense. When I first came to Israel in 1975, my Talmudic learning was entirely separate from my Aromatherapy practice. There appeared to be no connection between them, but since they were both essential aspects of my life, I wanted to learn what the Jewish tradition had to say about "Jewish Spiritual Aromatics." As I became more deeply immersed in my studies of Judaic Aromatics, I began to realize that the mystical and practical branches of my aromatic knowledge and experience were very closely inter-related. As I began to piece together fragments of ancient teachings from our various sources, I was amazed to find a multi-dimensional and unified treasure of deep wisdom. Jewish tradition is actually quite rich in aromatic discourse, and references to fragrance appear throughout the Torah and many holy texts. Yet, to reach the inner meaning of the words, and to arrive at a true and complete understanding of the Judaic point of view of this vitally important aspect of life, one must look deeply and put together many disparate pieces. The perspective gained is helpful for all who wish to reach a deeper understanding, regardless of one's religion or spiritual path.

Throughout my involvement in the field of Aromatherapy, I have discovered that very few people seem to know anything about holistic healing with natural fragrances. From the beginning, this lack of basic knowledge was very frustrating to me as a purveyor of botanical Essential Oils. In response to this problem, I decided to promote only the highest quality natural Organic and Wildcrafted Oils for health care, and set high standards for all of my products. When I first started out in 1982, my "Tiferet Aromatherapy" company was one of only three outlets selling natural essential oils to the retail market in the USA, while today there are over 3,000 companies offering them. I was primarily concerned that almost everyone seemed to be unaware of the vast differences between natural medicinal essential oils and toxic chemical fragrances. The companies selling the chemicals have tried "every trick in the book" to confuse the public into thinking that they are offering natural Oils, rather than synthetic fragrances which are now suspected to be carcinogenic in many instances. It seemed obvious that the most helpful way to resolve this confusion was through widespread education, so over the next thirty years I distributed over one million educational brochures, and lectured frequently across North America on various aspects of Aromatherapy health care.

As I began my studies of fragrance in Judaic literature several years after arriving in Israel, I would often bring a long list of my most pressing questions and topics of greatest interest to a rabbinical scholar for assistance and clarification. I soon discovered, to my surprise, that most Torah scholars seem to know very little - if anything - about what the Jewish sources have to say about fragrance. After many years of searching, I discovered that the key information is all there in small pieces scattered throughout the Judaic texts, but there apparently has been very little interest in piecing it together to build a meaningful understanding about the nature of fragrance, or the use of aromatic plants for healing purposes. Over thousands of years, very few Judaic books seem to have been written that are devoted to this area of study. Finally, after many years of digging below the surface of general knowledge, with the assistance of very diligent linguistic researchers exploring the ancient texts on my behalf, I have been able to decode, gather together and assemble the key aromatic teachings that are presented in this volume.

Perhaps what may be most remarkable of all is that the true "inside story" about fragrance has been so well hidden from most people for such a long time. How is it possible that so little attention has been paid to the sense of smell and the aromatic experience? Fragrance is an essential aspect of Jewish history and the vital lifeblood of our culture, from our heyday when the Temple stood and the transformative Incense filled the air, until the great day when the Anointing Oil will crown the Messiah! It is clearly the one sense that can be relied upon to give us accurate, unbiased information about what is really taking place in our environment and in the world that surrounds us. It is as if this greatest Secret of Life has been hidden away from us for two thousand years since the destruction of our Temple, until finally today we have been invited to take part in its rediscovery and revelation.

The unique and fascinating nature of this research and what it unveils to us regarding the true nature of aromatic medicine and holistic healing has inspired me to write this volume. Combining my training and experience in aromatherapy with the teachings I discovered in ancient

Jewish sources has allowed me to greatly expand and deepen my understanding of the function of fragrance and the use of aromatic plants in healing practice. In this two-part volume, I am excited to share with you the details I have learned of many mystical teachings that have deeply enriched my understanding of aromatherapy, along with the down-to-earth fundamental principles of fragrant healing practice that have emerged.

The convergence of theory and practice began to take form for me one day in 1990, when I was invited to meet Rabbi Menachem Burstein, the world's foremost scholar in the study of the botany, chemistry and aromatics of the First and Second Temples of Jerusalem. Rabbi Burstein heads an academy of Torah learning in Jerusalem that is devoted to this study. He had been working with his top students for the previous twenty-five years to precisely identify each of the eleven ingredients of the Temple incense. Although the Hebrew names of the ingredients are known, their exact botanical identities have been a topic of intense debate among the greatest Talmudic scholars over the past two thousand years.

Rabbi Burstein invited me to his office after a mutual friend had informed him of my work in aromatherapy, my love of high quality natural essential oils, and my ancient priestly lineage. He described his extensive study of the Temple incense, emphasizing the value of determining the exact identities of the spices, and the importance of smelling their true fragrances. At the time of our first meeting, Burstein had positively identified six of the eleven incense spices, and had carefully-researched speculations about the true identity of the other five, having narrowed down the possibilities to two or three for each spice.

At our meeting Rabbi Burstein suggested a special project. Since I am also a professional Perfumer, he advised me to build sets of natural essential oils of the Temple incense spices as their true identities became resolved, and to make these oils available to anyone and everyone, worldwide. He emphasized that while there is a strict Torah prohibition against attempting to make the incense with the various plant materials in their original form, there is no prohibition whatsoever against enjoying the fragrance of essential oil extracts of these same botanicals. In fact, doing so is very meritorious.

Rabbi Burstein strongly recommended that we all become familiar with the fragrances of the incense spices, to begin to "remind us of

Temple days." This, he explained, would help speed up the process of rebuilding the Temple. He also remarked that the presence of these fragrances in a person's home would be a *segula* (a blessing, or sign of good providence). The meeting was very inspiring, yet left me wondering how I would be able to positively identify the remaining five unknown spices, if he himself and his top scholars were unable to do so despite their vast knowledge and extensive research. The meeting with Rabbi Burstein inspired me to launch my own in-depth study of the Temple incense. I began to track down and import from around the world the essential oils of the incense spices that had been positively identified, as well as the Rabbi's candidates for the unresolved spices. My very first "Temple Incense Oils" sets were soon ready, but included only the six confirmed oils from among the eleven ingredients.

A few years later, I unexpectedly got an invitation to visit a Judean desert encampment to meet the "real Indiana Jones." Dr. Vendyl "Indiana" Jones is an extraordinary man. Global leader of the "B'nai Noah" organization of Righteous Gentiles, he was also an archaeologist *par excellence* who had been on a true-life search to locate the Ark of the Covenant and the treasures of the Temple, including, among other important artifacts, the actual Ark that was hidden away seven years before the destruction of the First Temple of Solomon. Vendyl's research over the past thirty-five years has focused on painstakingly deciphering the Copper Scroll of Jeremiah, produced and concealed at the same time that the Temple treasures were hidden. Dr. Jones' discovery in 1992 of 600 Kg. (1,320 lbs.) of ancient Temple incense, and a subsequent chemical analysis of this material, led to the positive identification of four of the five unresolved spices, allowing me to nearly complete my set of Temple Incense Oils.

Part One of this book includes remarkable mystical teachings about fragrance that I have culled from traditional Judaic sources, while **Part Two** illustrates some of the ways that my aromatic practice has developed, based on my training and experience combined with my scriptural studies, and details some unique practical applications of essential oils. Also featured in **Part Two** is background information about how Aromatherapy actually works as a sophisticated and powerful healing tool that can effectively treat all the levels of the body and soul simultaneously. My initial training with Patricia Davis at the London School of Aromatherapy, contact with other dynamic teachers and pioneers over the years, and day-to-day experience in aromatics over the past forty years have been influenced by my study of these ancient Judaic sources. At the heart of my current aromatherapy practice is an original fragrance testing technique that I have developed based on teachings from Genesis, which enables a practitioner to identify the correct essential oils to be used in any treatment, and their precise formulation. I have also decided to share my techniques by establishing an online school to offer personal training in aromatics. Information about the school can be found online at www.avaroma.com/training.php

Many thanks are due to the many excellent teachers and guides who have helped me along my way to see the hidden light and smell the roses. In particular I am deeply grateful for my inspiring studies with "Reb" Leah Golomb, helpful assistance from Rabbi Avraham Sutton, and supportive guidance from my long-time colleague, partner and friend, Aromatic Master John Steele of Lifetree Aromatix. I must also highly commend my wonderful early teachers including Patricia Davis and Beth Troy, among many others. Crucial editorial help and insightful teachings were kindly provided by Elana Schachter and Rabbi Sarah Etz Alon. I would also like to thank my extremely visionary publisher Santosh Krinsky of Lotus Press, who has given his support to my aromatherapy work for over twenty years, and to this project from its outset, always displaying incredible patience over many moons to see it through to completion.

I am very privileged to share with you in this volume some of the extraordinary artwork of Yitzhak ben Yehuda. Sixteen color plates of his large original oil paintings help to bring my Biblical stories to life. Born in Egypt and raised in Europe, Ben Yehuda has become a legendary artist in his own time. Upon his arrival in Israel in 1976, he turned his creative enthusiasm to painting Biblical narratives and landscapes of Israel. His work can be seen on his Website at www.benyehudastudio.com

This aromatic book is lovingly dedicated to the memory of our beautiful son Yacov Oren Yisrael haCohen, a holy warrior for peace who cherished the earth, and always had a kind word and a smile, even throughout the most difficult times.

Avraham Sand
Moshav Me'or Modi'im, Israel
December, 2011

The Fragrance of the Garden of Eden

Foreword to "Mystical Aromatherapy"

"Mystical Aromatherapy" is a book to delight every one of our senses, focusing on the most important, the oldest and the littlest known of them, our sense of smell. It is said that when the Messiah comes he will know each of us by our fragrance.

Besides his other talents, Avraham Sand has the special gift of being an excellent teacher, so he is able to explain to us in simple terms the significance of the spices of the Ketoret, the Incense Offering of the Temple for God. He is able to bring back alive for us the ancient teachings about this mystical fragrance, so we can understand it again in its depth and beauty from the past, and how to better welcome this special blend of spices when it returns to our world in the future.

I have known Avraham and his family for more than 20 years, and have watched as he and his wife Leah put all the pieces of this hidden puzzle together for us, how to access the benefit of pure Essential Oils in our lives right now.

Today there are many competitors for our olfactory glands (those special organs that determine our sense of smell), and most of them are coming from synthetic sources. These chemicals are very harmful to us, and are found in modern personal care products, cleaning aids and laundry soaps, and there is even new evidence emerging from scientific studies that synthetic fragrances are actually changing our DNA (not to our benefit), accelerating disease, infertility and needless suffering.

This is why Avraham's book has arrived just in time, to teach us about the deeper knowledge and understanding of how to incorporate natural fragrances in our daily lives. This brings us to a place of solid practical knowledge to learn how to use the purest of essential oils for healing and joy, helping us to move forward into a most beautiful, healthy and fragrant future.

Shoshanna Harrari
Moshav Ramat Raziel, Israel
Author of "The Seven Healing Fruits of Israel"
and "The Garden of Spices"

Shoshanna Harrari is highly praised throughout Israel and internationally, thanks to her extensive knowledge and experience as a Master healer, herbalist, harpist, chef and dietary specialist.

Highly Aromatic Comments

by John Steele

Mystical Aromatherapy is an important contribution to understanding the depth and profound meaning of the holy tradition of smell and fragrance in ancient Israel. The combination of this ancient wisdom with modern aromatherapy/sacred healing creates an integrated aromatic paradigm of great value. Avraham Sand weaves together references from the Bible, the Talmud the Kabala, commentary from learned rabbis, botanists and archaeologists (including the original Indiana Jones) plus his own experience as a perfumer and Judaic fragrance researcher, into a holistic fragrant tapestry.

A fascinating central theme of the book is the Scent of Paradise, "the most beautiful fragrance in the world," which emanates from the Garden of Eden. This primeval Scent of Paradise was saturated in the aromatic garments of Creation that Adam and Eve wore. These garments were sewn together into a single vest of power (the *Meil Hatzedaka*) and passed on to their son Seth and then through the Biblical lineage of Noah, Abraham. Isaac, Jacob and Moses. This Scent of Paradise is also found in the Temple Incense, the Anointing Oil of the Temple, the Messiah and the Cave of the Patriarchs.

Sand shows that the sacred use of fragrance unites heaven and earth, the spiritual and the physical as well as the conscious mind and the intuition. The undefiled sense of olfactory wisdom that we inherited from the Garden of Eden is a key thread throughout this thought provoking book, which will be of interest to researchers of the spiritual dimension of aromatic history and to contemporary practitioners of sacred aromatic healing based on what Sand refers to as "primordial aromatherapy."

About John Steele:

John is a fragrance designer for his company Lifetree Aromatix, which offers rare organic essential oils and exotic floral absolutes to a discerning clientele. He enjoys communicating his passion for the spiritual use of aromatic plants in ancient civilizations and shamanic cultures. He graduated from UC Berkeley with studies in English literature, archaeology and anthropology. Further doctoral research was focused on an interdisciplinary study of memory. At the University of London he was a visiting lecturer in General Systems Theory.

John has served on the board of the American Aromatherapy Association and consulted on future trends in aromatherapy for the Aveda Corporation. He has also lectured for the American Society of Perfumers, the Fragrance Foundations Summit 2000, the Pacific Institute of Aromatherapy, the Bowers Museum and UC Berkeley. John also has given several presentations on The Mysteries of Smell and Fragrance in Ancient Israel.

He is a co-author, with Paul Devereux and David Kubrin of Earthmind (Harper and Row, 1989), an exploration of the Gaia hypothesis that the Earth is a living super organism. He also contributed a chapter on "The Sacred Use of Fragrance in Amazonian Shamanism" to the Smell Culture Reader (Berg, 2006, ed. J.Drobnick).

Key to Color Plates

16 Color Photos of Original Oil Paintings
by Yitzhak Ben Yehuda

1. Jacob's Dream. A man who fathered the twelve Tribes of Israel is overtaken by a profound sleep. The vistas of the future are revealed to him, such as the various nations that will rise and fall against Israel, and the future Temple. The billows that look like cloud in this painting depict the angels ascending to heaven and descending, as they journey to and fro.
2. Vision of Rachel. The woman of valor who channels all prayers to the Throne of Glory. Her tomb (depicted) near Bethlehem is a holy place, where women from throughout the world congregate, to insure that their supplications will be answered.
3. Vision of Rachael #2. This version includes the Hebrew poem of the ancient "Woman of Valor" of King Solomon (Proverbs).
4. The Tree of Life. Encompassed by the mystical spheres which uphold the universe, husband and wife stand hand-in-hand in the Garden of Eden.
5. Moses. The man of God had utter and complete humility when he received the Divine Law. He is known as the greatest Prophet of all time to the people of Israel.
6. The Great Day at Sinai. Moses in a state of transformation, as he approaches the Divine Presence to receive the Torah, the basis of Jewish Law and worldwide monotheistic practice. Prior to the Revelation, the world was filled with thunder, lightning and fire, which gave way to the still small voice which became visible in the inscriptions written upon the two tablets.
7. 'Reb' Shlomo portrait. A brilliant and righteous man who personally befriended and uplifted hundreds of thousands of souls as a gentle giant of love, scripture and song.
8. 'Reb' Shlomo mosaic. The great selfless soul Rabbi Shlomo Carlebach, an illustrious teacher of our generation who lived for the world we will build tomorrow.

9. The Oak of Abraham. A symbolic painting of cousins, a Jew and two Moslems, conversing in mutual respect under the shadow of their common forefather, Abraham.

10. The Sacrifice of Isaac. The epitome of an act that required the ultimate degree of devotion, faith and trust in the Will of the Holy One.

11. Jerusalem. The holy city of peace, dreams and hope.

12. The Youth David. The youngest of seven brothers, he was assigned to tend the family flock. Soon afterwards he would be crowned the King of Israel.

13. Jerusalem Pilgrimage Festival. Three times during the year in the days of the Temple, many people would ascend to Jerusalem to bring their gifts of peace.

14. The High Priest. The crowning glory of sanctity and purity.

15. The High Priest #2. He alone was designated to offer the Temple incense inside the Holy of Holies on Yom Kippur.

16. The Sea of Galilee. The village of Tiberias, as it might have looked in the days of the Temple.

17. The Desert Tabernacle. Courtesy of Vendyl Jones Research Center.

18. The Tabernacle at Gilgal. Courtesy of Vendyl Jones Research Center.

Chapter 1

Aromatic Elements of Creation

In our holy Jewish tradition, we learn that all of the natural botanical plants were brought into the world on the third day of creation to bring forth food for sustenance and medicine to treat every sickness and disease. They were compassionately set in place to be ready for the animals and people that were created later, on the sixth day, who would rely upon them to maintain life and health. The highly aromatic and medicinal varieties are among the original plants of the Garden of Eden, which were later scattered to the four corners of the earth.[1] In fact the Hebrew word for "fragrances" – *Bisamim* - is the same as the word meaning "in heaven" – *baShamayim* - but with different vowel points.

The rather obscure teachings concerning aromatics are first alluded to in the Biblical story of creation at the very beginning of the holy Torah ("5 Books of Moses"), where the events that transpired in the "Garden of Eden," also known as "paradise," are described. Other revelations in the Torah, transmitted in its entirety to Moses on Mt. Sinai, delve deeper into the secrets of aromatics, in the detailed descriptions of the Temple Incense and the Anointing Oil, the epitome of Judaic Aromatherapy. These divine formulas were used as sacraments during the exodus from Egypt, during the time of Solomon's Temple and the Second Temple of Jerusalem, and they will hopefully be employed again in the Third Temple soon to come. The revelations of the true nature and scope of Aromatics culminate in the Jewish concept of the future "Messiah" (in Hebrew "*Mashiach,*" meaning the "Anointed one"), who will arrive at the "End of Days" and judge by his sense of smell.[2] Detailed information about the Messiah is presented at the end of Chapter 4.

All of our senses are mentioned in the creation story, except the sense of smell. According to this teaching, all of our senses fell to a lower spiritual level when Adam and Eve tragically ate the forbidden fruit of the Tree of Knowledge, which in part led to our expulsion from the Garden. We learn that only our *Sense of Smell* was not involved in the "original sin," since it was not mentioned in the story. That one sense has always remained holy. Shortly after man was expelled from the Garden, he requested permission to briefly re-enter to collect vital aromatic plants that we would need for healing and renewal, and to aid us in making our way back to the Garden forever. The special aromatic plants that Man collected included the spices that would be needed to make the Temple incense, which would bring great joy to the Holy One.

Thus our potential connection with the fragrant medicinal plants of the Garden of Eden, as can be revealed through our highly elevated sense of smell, remains intact today. We actually still have this special gift, whenever we make use of it. According to Jewish tradition, one primary result of being expelled from the Garden has been that our other senses are involved with the mundane world in a way that can easily bring confusion and ill health, but **our olfactory ability is still potentially as pure today as it was when it was first created.** Thus fragrance still has the power to transport us through vast spans of time, even to past lifetimes, and to trigger vivid memories. It is also the most reliable channel to guide us to the aromatic medicines we need for optimal health.

Understanding that our sense of smell is totally reliable has taught me to implicitly trust this special intuitive ability, as I have learned to observe and use it effectively. It has led to the development of my own fragrance testing technique that I employ very effectively in aromatherapy practice, and teach to my students. This method relies upon and demonstrates the consistent aromatic ability of the person receiving the treatment to accurately select the fragrant medicine(s) to be used, and their precise formulation. The details of my technique are presented in Chapter 8.

When the Jewish people left Egypt in 1240 BCE on their way to the land of Israel, upon their departure they were given "gifts" by the Egyptians. One may assume that these treasures included an array of medicines and sacraments: precious gums, aromatic herbs and spices, herbal extracts, and essential oils produced by a solar still. All of these were among the most precious commodities of ancient Egyptian culture. The priestly Jewish tribe of Levi, including the family of *Cohanim* – Priests - were never enslaved by the Egyptians. When Joseph was second-in-command under Pharaoh in Egypt, he was careful not to tax the priestly clans, thus setting the precedent that these families would also not be taxed by hard labor and enslaved, as were the rest of the Jewish people.

Since they were free to pursue their own interests, and in order to meet the needs of the community, some of the Levites and Priests became highly trained by the Egyptian experts in alchemy, herbal medicine, natural cosmetology and embalming. They ultimately took this knowledge and their medications along on the journey to the Holy Land. At Mt. Sinai, Moses received recipes and instructions for producing the Temple Incense and the Anointing Oil, putting many of these aromatic materials to sacred use.

Every civilized culture for thousands of years has practiced the ancient arts of healing, rejuvenation and even embalming with natural herbal botanicals and their extracts. The first synthetic fragrances and medicines were developed only within the past 100 years. Before then, and throughout history, every great doctor was a master herbalist, and botanical medications were employed in every household. Each ancient culture has incorporated botanical usage, history and religious practice in unique ways, and left extensive records, fully documenting the successful use of herbal medicine. There are also ongoing traditions of holistic practice, especially in the Orient, based on the transmission of knowledge that has stayed intact over thousands of years.

By comparison, modern medicine has made miraculous discoveries and sweeping advances in the understanding and treatment of many severe health-threatening conditions. However, the modern approach has increasingly become very symptom-oriented, often overlooking or misunderstanding the deeper root causes of ailment, imbalance and disease. In the very best medical schools today there may be very little - if any - training in herbal medicine, or other long-proven holistic healing techniques such as acupuncture. There is a lack of true understanding and emphasis regarding proper diet and exercise. In particular, herbs and their derivatives, the true God-given medicines of the ages with long track-records of success, may tend to be overlooked in training, and not regarded as an important aspect of medical education. Thus the basis of all former health maintenance, medical treatment, along with virtually all of the medicines that have been so successfully employed throughout the world over the past few thousand years, has recently been largely dismissed by today's medical establishment.

As a result, it should come as no surprise that our modern medical doctors are incapable of effectively treating common everyday ailments such as a cold, flu or headache. Without any real knowledge of herbs, most common everyday conditions can simply not be treated effectively, and will not just "go away." The synthetic pharmaceutical medicines that doctors prescribe, supporting the multi-billion dollar drug industry, are little more than a "band aid" approach, usually addressing the symptoms and not the underlying causes of ailment. These largely unproven laboratory-made chemicals that we know as "modern medicine" often further aggravate our overall health condition. While some symptoms may disappear, others may appear in their place, simply because the true underlying problem has not been properly diagnosed or treated.

Natural aromatics of various types were one of the earliest, most important and valuable trade materials of the ancient world. Specialized caravans traveled famous spice routes, bringing the finest rare and highly prized spices to Egypt and Europe from the East. In classic Biblical stories, Jacob [*Color Plate 1 – Jacob's Dream*] carried perfumes which may have inspired his famous dream. The son of Jacob and Rachel [*Color Plates 2 and 3 – Vision of Rachel*], Joseph "the Righteous," was sold by his brothers and carried off to Egypt by a caravan of perfume merchants transporting aromatic herbs, various types of plant extracts, and pleasant smelling aromatic oils. The Torah teaches that this was arranged by the Holy One to spare Joseph from offensive and unpleasant odors. Usually such caravans carried vile smelling turpentine, tar and other foul-smelling materials.

Mordechai, the Purim hero, is alluded to in the written Torah where *Mor Dror* - pure myrrh - for the Anointing Oil is mentioned. According to the famous Torah commentator Rashi, this pure myrrh is the *Rosh Besamim* – the chief of all the spices. The righteous men of the Great Assembly are compared to the spices, and their leader was also named Mordechai. The classical commentator Onkelos calls this spice "*Mari Dachya*" – Aramaic for pure myrrh, which has the same letters as MoRDeChaY. Our hero Mordechai was the leader of all the righteous people of his generation, and he worked to "finely grind" Haman and his ten sons who were completely nullified. This relates to the property of myrrh in the Anointing Oil: it nullifies evil.

The Sages enthusiastically praised the value of fragrances for the Jewish ceremony performed at the end of the Sabbath known as *Habdallah*

– Separation - which brings in the new week on Saturday night. In this ceremony we experience and bless God for a sweet fragrance which lifts our spirits to console and fortify us for the loss of our *Neshama Yetirah* – our "extra Soul." Then we bless the candle light, as we allow our "extra soul" to leave through our fingernails, until the following Sabbath. Other sources say that during the Sabbath the "fires of the underworld" are quiet, but when the Sabbath ends, the fires are lit again, and the soul needs relief from this foul odor.

One must use only a pleasant natural fragrance that requires a blessing for the ceremony. It is not permissible to make a blessing on the common synthetic chemical fragrances. The sages say that those who engage in acts of self-sacrifice, making themselves humble and nullifying their ego to privately or publicly sanctify the Holy One, raise up a heavenly fragrance. As a person reaches a higher spiritual level, they ultimately begin to emanate a scent that more and more resembles the aroma of paradise, none other than the sacred fragrance of the Temple, imbued with incense.

The Dynamics of Creation

"In the beginning, the Holy One created worlds and destroyed them" [*Bereshit Raba 3:7*]. Most of the vessels of these worlds were purposely shattered by God seven times during the initial stages of creation. When He allowed tiny bits of His infinite Light to shine into them, each vessel burst into minute particles and fell, forming the basis for lower, more physical worlds. Finally the material universe that we live in today came into existence. The Tree of Life [*Color Plate 4 – Tree of Life*] depicts 11 "*Sefirot*" (singular, "*Sefira*") – which symbolize divine vessels, the basic modalities that are the true building blocks of life. Only the lower seven *Sefirot* of the Tree were shattered in the initial stages of creation, while the four upper *Sefirot* remained intact.

These 11 basic life energies perfectly correspond to the 11 Spices of the *Ketoret* - the **Temple Incense** which was carefully compounded by master craftsmen from a sacred and detailed recipe. The incense formula and its mystical secrets were fully revealed to Moses [*Color Plate 5 – Moses*] on Mount Sinai [*Color Plate 6 – The Great Day at Sinai*] as a part of the transmission of our Holy Torah. The 4 major incense spices - those that correspond with the four upper *Sefirot* which remained intact during the stages of Creation - comprise nearly 80% of the mixture, and these 4 are mentioned in the written Torah. The other

7 Spices which correspond with the lower seven *Sefirot* that shattered are mentioned only in the Oral Law.

The 11 spices were ground into a very fine and well-mixed powder. Grinding the Temple Incense represents the seven times that the vessels shattered during the initial stages of Creation. Fine grinding causes the fragrance of the spices to be enriched and dispersed, as tiny droplets of essential oil are released. This grinding of the mixture, accompanied by a voice chanting rhythmically, is what actually gave the incense its special mystical powers of Life-over-Death, and the ability to lift a person to the highly exalted state of consciousness known as *Nevuah* ("Prophecy").[3]

The Creation of Man

In the Creation story, God said: "Let *Us* make Man with our image and likeness"[4] and this Voice was instilled in the Universe. This is the only place in the Creation story where the plural form is used. God took counsel, so to speak, and wanted the Angels, all of the worlds and the entire universe to contribute their will and desire to the mission of designing Man. It was a group project in which, ultimately, *almost all* of God's creation participated. Also, God wanted Man to attain all Worlds, and be the connecting link between them. Adam was designed to contain all souls. In other words, the Creator wanted each dimension of existence to give something of itself to Man. In this way, each dimension would have a natural compassion for him.

The intention of the Holy One, from the beginning, was to place Man in a spiritually rich and rewarding environment where he would be able to live a fruitful spiritual life forever. God prepared a template with which He would now shape Man, and give him an intellect and the power of understanding [Rashi]. One primary distinction between Man and the rest of creation that demonstrates that Man was created in the image of God is the Divine gift of free will [Sforno]. Thus Man alone has the ability to guide his actions through his reasoning and intellect [Rambam]. God wanted all of creation to be tied to Man's actions, for better or for worse. This included a Heavenly partnership agreement that if Man lived righteously, according to God's will, all of creation would have joy from him; but if, by misfortune, Man would sin, cause a blemish, or create disorder in any of these dimensions, every Angel and world would ask for Mercy on his behalf.[5]

Only the *Sitra Achra* - the "Other Side" - the Evil inclination, also known as samaEl, the Angel of Death, and the parasitic forces of evil which live off mankind's sins refused to participate. They refused to give their energy to the project of creating Man. If they had co-operated, this world would have been created perfectly from the very beginning, and remained absolutely perfect throughout all eternity. There would be no *klipa* - shell - surrounding existence.[6] As a result of their refusal to participate in Man's creation, when God and the Universe created Man, the Other Side was left out, and thus fell down to the lower level of this world. He was transformed into a snake, to constantly contend against Man. Instead of giving life force and support to Man, evil always wants the opposite.

"Jealousy, lust and (the pursuit of) honor/glory remove a person from the world."[7] The ministering Angels said before the Holy One, "Master of the Worlds! What is Man that you would even consider him? His life will be nothing but vanity. He won't even be able to control his own desires!" The Holy One replied, "Just as you praise Me in Heaven above, Man will praise Me on earth below. And furthermore, can you know the inner essence of all My creatures? Can you stand before Me and give names to them?" They stood but were unable to do so. Immediately Adam stood and gave names to all the animals, indicating that he had the ability to master all physical forces, and unlike the Angels, he was a composite of all of them. Seeing this, the evil Angels, who fell because of their jealousy, took council among themselves saying, "We must make sure than Man will sin before his Creator now, or else we will never be able to overcome him."[8]

Now *samaEl* was a very great minister in heaven, having 12 wings, indicating a very exalted level before his fall. He descended with his legions, and beheld each of the creatures that the Holy One had created. Not one was wise enough to commit evil except the nachash – the snake - as it is written, "The Snake was more subtle/sneaky than all the beasts that God had made."[9] In the same way that a person can be possessed by an evil spirit, all that the snake did and all that it said was being controlled by *samaEl*.[10]

According to Rav Chaim Vital, this fall happened in order to prevent the evil forces from receiving direct nourishment from the holy life force in heaven above. The Holy One caused them to descend, until the time when "Death (meaning the Angel of Death and his evil legions) will be swallowed up forever, and *HaShem Elokim* (the Great Spirit) will wipe the tears off every face. He will remove the insult against His people from the entire world, as He has declared."[11] In the meantime, because he refused to contribute his portion to humanity, and having lost his exalted status, Evil is constantly trying to trip people and cause them to sin. Angered that he himself was cast down to this lower world, the Other Side is on a mission to bring Man down with him to a lower level, in every way he can, and he has no mercy.

Thus on the very first day of their life, the first man and first woman transgressed. As a result, they were severely punished, banished from Paradise, and condemned to struggle against the forces of evil, working hard to sustain themselves in a material world. The snake poisoned Chava, and consequently Adam, by seducing them to eat the forbidden fruit. Man was clearly created with the flaw of a tendency to sin, but he was also given the ability to overcome this built-in flaw to attain his own perfection. Even, or perhaps especially, when he does wrong, the Holy One comes to his assistance and judges him mercifully. This is beyond the capacity of the Angels.

While the divine soul seeks and yearns to be united with the Holy One, its source of life, the animal soul is only interested in self-gratification. The divine soul sees itself as included in and dissolving into the One-ness of the Great Spirit, while the animal soul sees itself as a separate entity, concerned only with its own needs and desires. These two kingdoms are constantly struggling, each wanting to completely rule over the other. This is the ongoing struggle that takes place within each one of us every day, except for the rare individual that is either completely righteous or completely wicked.

These evil forces can continue to exist only by causing human beings to fall, then parasitically sucking the life-force from them. After Adam sinned, his stature greatly diminished and all of the exalted levels that had been given to him (on loan) quickly departed from him. As a result, he descended, and was forced to clothe himself in a coarse physical body. Initially, Adam and Chava were clothed in garments of Light. Only after they sinned did God make them garments of skin/hide, the skin of the snake.[12] According to the interpretation of Rabbi Meir, these were garments of Light. Because of the *Sitra Achra*, man was given a levush - a garment - the body, and a klipa – a shell, or protective layer, and this left man with a deep impurity known as "*zehuma,*" that brings death and decay into this world. In fact the distinctively different foul odors which emanate from various states of zehuma reveal exact and reliable information to a trained aromatherapist regarding the state of a person's health. Based on this principle, doctors throughout the world for thousands of years have been able to accurately diagnose an ailment or condition based on the specific fragrance of their client.

Surprisingly, we are not actually meant to destroy the animal soul or completely do away with the *Yetzer haRa* – the evil inclination. Instead, it is our task to educate and uplift it by being *b'simcha tamid* - always joyous, so that the evil inclination will join with the Divine Soul in serving God, completing this world and making it a dwelling place for the *Shechina* – the Divine Presence. We will continue to struggle until "Death will be swallowed up forever" at the "End of Days," which will herald the arrival of the Messiah.[13]

After falling down to this world, the Other Side also became known as "The Angel of Death." However, when Moses ascended Mt. Sinai generations later, through his good deeds he merited to receive a divine gift from this dark Angel: the "secret of secrets" regarding the miraculous life-saving properties of the Temple Incense. When Moses went up to heaven to receive the Torah, he was representing Primordial Man. It was as if it was still the time before Man had been fully created. On this occasion the Other Side changed his mind. He was so inspired by Moses that he finally decided to co-operate in Man's creation. Thus he gave Man the antidote to death by revealing the secret of the Incense to Moses: that it is in fact the original "Rescue Remedy" of life ruling over death.

Just as Adam contained all souls within himself, Moses was equivalent to all of Israel. When Adam's soul reincarnated as Moses, through the power of his deeds he regained Adam's highest levels of consciousness. Moses reached the very highest consciousness level (sometimes referred to as the "forty-ninth gate") when he received the Torah, the highest revelation of supernal wisdom, distilled, condensed and compacted enough to be accessible to humans.[14]

Thus Moses was found to be more worthy than Adam. While the Evil One did not support Adam, he willingly gave a portion of his own life-force to Moses, because Adam had done nothing to deserve the exalted levels that were loaned to him. They were all a gift, and were not earned. In contrast, Moses built himself up by his own efforts and good deeds. Because of this, the Evil one also contributed. This was the case because the Evil one, also called Satan (the Accuser), is really an aspect of God's own attribute of Justice, which requires that Man deserve the good that he is given. Thus Moses was taught the mystery of the Ketoret by none other than the Angel of Death.

The Garden of Eden was Paradise and had the most beautiful fragrance in the world. Man and woman were originally in an absolutely perfect state of radiant health and high consciousness. According to our holy tradition, Adam and Eve had access to the primordial Light of Creation during their first 36 hours of life.[15] This light allowed them to see from one end of the world to the other, and throughout all time. In the beginning, all of our senses were on the same level as the Soul, but when they participated in eating the forbidden fruit, the senses descended to the "body" level - all *except the Sense of Smell*, which did not participate in the sin. Our ethereal, spiritual body then coarsened, and we were given a body of flesh and bones. The primordial light was then stored away for the righteous ones in the future.

When the first woman and man ate fruit from the forbidden Tree of Knowledge, they damaged our ability to eat in holiness, for all future generations until the End of Days. Since then, every act of eating has included some impurity and waste. In fact, illness and death came from this primordial error. The resulting impurity can be partly repaired by fasting, but it is primarily fixed by learning how to eat properly. According to our teacher, Rabbi Shlomo Carlebach of Blessed memory [*Color Plates 7 and 8 – Reb Shlomo*], we were not expelled from the Garden simply because we ate the forbidden fruit. That mistake could have been rectified without such serious consequences. We actually fell from grace and were thrown out when Adam blamed his wife (and God!) for giving him the wrong food.

Thus man's most crucial repair has been to learn to "cover" for his wife, and especially *not to blame her* – even when she makes a mistake. Also, since the woman had a share in this tragic error by blaming the snake instead of taking responsibility upon herself, she also must learn to "cover" for her partner and not blame him. Another powerful repair of the first sin for a woman is learning to offer the right food to her partner. Many men may also have to learn to build (actually, to rebuild) trust that the woman in their life is offering them the right food.[16]

In the fall of our senses, man lost his initial holiness, and then had to be dressed in the garments of a material body to cover and protect his divine soul: "We find that the inner being (the soul) is the true self, while the body is merely a garment with which the soul covers itself while (sojourning) in this world. At the moment of death, when the soul departs (and with it the sense of smell, the last active sense), this garment is removed, and (the soul) is clothed in a pure, clean, spiritual garment (which is the spiritual energy which surrounds the soul when it re-enters the Garden)... Just as a tailor makes a suit of clothes to fit a person's physique, so (does) the Holy One make the body as a garment to clothe the soul...(and the body is made) according to the pattern of the soul."[17]

Primordial Roots of Aromatherapy

Our Rabbis point out that our sense of smell is the only one of our five senses that is *not specifically mentioned* as having been involved in the primordial sin of eating from the Tree of Knowledge, in the verses at the beginning of Genesis. Eve "listened" to the snake, "saw" the good fruit, "touched" and "tasted" it. There is no mention of smelling the fruit or any reference to fragrance at all. The Garden of Eden was the headquarters of the most beautiful aroma on earth, the most divine fragrance in all of Creation, and this sense is conspicuous by its very absence in the Creation story. It never became corrupted or fell to a lower level of consciousness, as our other senses did. From this our Rabbis declare that our sense of smell is still potentially as pure and holy today as it was in the Garden of Eden. It has remained and will remain forever a pure soul experience. In fact, our sense of smell is the most elevated aspect of our being, and it is **the primary vehicle of our enlightened super-consciousness, which is known as *Ruach HaKodesh*** ("Holy Spirit").[18]

This teaching finds a striking validation in a biological examination of the human body. All our other senses go through a complex processing system before any information enters and is encoded in the "rational brain," the cortical memory center, otherwise known as the hippocampus. In contrast, our sense of smell has a direct "hotline" pathway to the higher "limbic brain" area, and it is much more trustworthy than our other senses. Only 3 neurons connect the nose to the outer layer of the brain, known as the cortex. The limbic brain is the cerebral area that is associated with dreams, intuition and higher consciousness, in addition to its involvement with our sense of smell. Most of its functions are still a mystery. However, it does seem that the limbic brain is where the soul and body connect. Our sense of smell elevates the physical to the spiritual, as matter touches the soul and enlightens it in a way that by-passes our lower pleasure centers. In this process of surrendering our rational mind to our higher consciousness, we also uplift our ego to a pure fragrance that enters into God's Divine Being and brings Joy, in the same way that the primary function of the Temple Incense is to bring Joy to the Holy One.[19]

The rational part of our brain can easily make mistakes. We don't have all of the information, we don't see the whole picture, and we can become confused. Our rational thinking process may often be distorted and unreliable. The limbic brain however is like a "third eye" - it may be more open or more closed – but it is free from the pitfall of confusing things the way our rational brain can. As a function of our Holy Spirit, our sense of smell can be trained, and ultimately trusted, to give us accurate and reliable information whenever called upon.

"**Aromatherapy**" is a term which is often mistakenly thought to imply a **therapy** treatment using **Aroma**. This is not really the most accurate meaning or understanding. Practically speaking, the healing treatment *might* – or *might not* – include a fragrant experience involving the nose and olfactory system. The overall healing effect however is not necessarily experienced by smelling the aroma, although this is often an important component, especially in influencing the mind, emotions and Spirit.

A more accurate understanding of the term "Aromatherapy" might be this: experiencing the **Aroma** of a natural substance *enables the body to very accurately detect* whether or not this aromatic substance is the proper healing **therapy** that the body needs. The most helpful medicine for each person is accurately revealed by his or her personal sensory response to the aroma of the plant or its derivatives. Simply put, the more a person is drawn to a fragrance, the more effective it will be as a component *in any form* of healing and rebalancing treatment. Conversely, when a person is *not drawn* to a fragrance, especially if they are repelled by it, that fragrance should absolutely be *avoided* – regardless of any theoretical information that would recommend it. This is the true key to safe, effective, and professional aromatherapy practice.

Being drawn to a fragrance is an intuitive experience – we like it because we need it. *Not* liking a fragrance is a warning to not repeat the

Primordial Sin: taking into the body a substance that is not good for it. *Our sense of smell, since it is still attached to our higher self, constantly protects us by drawing us closer to the things we need for health and survival, while repelling us from things of ill-health and danger.* This special protective ability is activated not only by aromatic plants and food, but also by our intuitive response to other people and physical surroundings. Intuitively, we know what is healthy for us and what to avoid. Our sense of smell is at the very center of this protective guidance system. As our teacher Rabbi Shlomo Carlebach once said, "When you don't know what to do or which way to go... if it smells like Shabbos ("the Sabbath"), go for it!"

When a person is ill, he will have *Ruach HaKodesh* ("Holy Spirit") through his sense of smell. The body in its ideal state is complete and healthy. When something is broken, the body intuitively knows what it needs. A person's sense of smell reaches to this perfect place, where his body and soul connect. Smell is the purest, most direct means to assist in the connection and integration of body and soul. Thus, when we smell a natural aromatic medicine, from the fragrance response of our Holy Spirit, we quickly become aware of whether or not that element is missing in our chemistry. Our sense of smell is very carefully and accurately checking for the missing link.

When we become ill, a limb, organ or body function breaks down, and that broken place is sending out a distress signal through our higher consciousness and sensory systems. Thus, when we smell the medicine we need, we can quickly and easily identify it. Finding one's true remedy requires personal aromatic experience. *A healer can offer suggestions or "candidates," but the definitive choice(s) about the best medicine(s) to use, those that will truly help the most,* ***must come from the person seeking the healing.***

Chapter 2

Fragrant Stories of the Bible

The Aromatic Garment of the Garden of Eden

God made special garments for Adam and Eve that were imbued with the heavenly fragrance of Eden. When he was first created, man was pure and holy, and was asked to keep only one commandment: do not eat from the Tree of Knowledge. After this edict was violated, the possibility of evil and sexual temptation came into the world, and man began to have a *Yetzer haRa* – an evil urge. Clothing was then needed, primarily to help bring sexual passion under control. The Torah considers the individual who can completely control his sexual desires as one who can control all of his emotions, and reach spiritual perfection.

After eating from the Tree of Knowledge, the Torah tells us, "The eyes of both of them were opened, and they knew that they were naked. They sewed fig leaves and made themselves loincloths." [Genesis 3:7] A Hebrew word for garment - *levoosh* – comes from the root word *boosha* – shame, indicating that one reason for wearing clothing is shame. Another Hebrew word for garment is *boged* – to rebel, which indicates that another reason why we wear clothing is because man rebelled against God. This does not imply that sexuality is something that is inherently evil, from the Judaic perspective. The Torah views sex as something beautiful and pleasurable, and as the act that does the most to strengthen the bond between husband and wife. At the same time, the Torah recognizes that when misused, sex can be the most destructive and debilitating force in the world. From all this, we see that clothing functions as a balancing force against improper sexual desires.[1]

God understood the need for spiritual and physical protection after Adam and Eve were ejected from the Garden. He saw that they found no satisfaction in the fig leaves they had sewn together, so He made more permanent garments for them: "God made garments of (leather) skins for Adam and his wife, and He clothed them."[2] According to one Midrash, the garments were made from the skin of the Snake that tempted Eve to eat the forbidden fruit, while other opinions say that they were crafted from the skin of the rainbow-colored unicorn that

God made for the coverings of the Tabernacle.[3]

These garments were later sewn together into a one-piece vestment known as the *Meil Hatzedaka* – the "Garment of the Balancing Force," which was always highly treasured, and carefully preserved for future generations. It is described in later Kabbalistic writings as a hooded, sleeveless deer skin that draped over the bearer's shoulders and chest, down to the navel, and fell along the sides of the loins. This revered and powerful mantle was colorfully painted or engraved with divine names, designs of animals, mystical symbols and invocations, and it was imbued with the magnificent fragrance of the Garden of Eden.

Whoever wore it had the power to subdue all beasts, which refers not only to its ability to aid in hunting, but also its ability to help balance sexual forces, and to guide one in mastering one's own animal nature. Not only was the person who wore it empowered with supernatural abilities, but the mysterious garment itself wielded the power to alter the ordinary. Accounts dating as early as the ninth century BCE allude to a continual "thread" which resurfaces many times in the Biblical stories that follow Adam's expulsion from the Garden.[4]

In part, the attributes of the deer - passion and zealousness - were invested in the Garment.[5] We are taught that passion is the essential divine life-force of all living things, while hesitation and lack of passion are the antithesis of the mystic path.[6] Deerskin is also special because "it does not cling to its flesh,"[7] implying that a deer is a spirit animal that is not as fully manifested in the physical realm as most other creatures. The mystic needs to walk in the realms of both spirit and matter, while attached to neither, and thus benefits from donning deer skin. The idea of skin wielding supernal powers is not confined to discussions about the garment of the balancing force. The skin in ancient Hebrew cosmology is the seat of the aura of divine light that enables the existence of any living thing.[8]

Adam and Eve bore children, and chose to transmit this divine gift as a special initiation only to those who truly merited to receive it. They gave it to their son Seth, and it was passed down through successive generations to Noah, who took the garment into the Ark. One tradition says that the garment was later passed down to our patriarch Abraham, who donned it when he brought his son Isaac to Mt. Moriah to be sacrificed. Another tradition says that Ham, Noah's son, received the garment and then gave it to the wicked King Nimrod, and that

Esav killed Nimrod to obtain it.[9] He gave the garment to his mother Rebecca to store, and she used it to disguise Jacob, which empowered him to obtain Isaac's blessing. Later, Jacob endowed this legendary vestment to Joseph, and it became known as the "coat of many colors." The brothers dipped a fragment of it in blood and presented it to their father to imply that Joseph had been attacked by wild animals, and it was later grabbed by Potiphar's wife. It would continue to be ceremoniously passed down from prophet to prophet, and was mentioned in many biblical stories such as those of Elijah and his disciple Elisha. Just before the destruction of Solomon's Temple, the prophet Jeremiah finally placed the garment inside in the Ark of the Covenant, where it remains to this day, for safekeeping until the Third Temple.[10]

Tradition is clear that the aromatic mantle that Adam wore when he left the Garden of Eden is the same garment worn by Elijah the Prophet. The transmission of this vestment in part went through Noah, Abraham, Isaac, Jacob, Joseph, Moses, Joshua, Elijah and Elisha. Because the Garment carried the specific attribute of mediating the elements of Creation, it is logical that it would be infused with the aromatic essence of the Garden, because Air is the mediating element. Since the Aroma of an object expresses its essence, the Aromatic Garment emanates the very essence of the Garden of Eden, the primal essence of Creation itself, and it reflects the Mind of the Holy Blessed One at the time of Creation.[11]

The Cave of the Patriarchs[12]

In the Garden of Eden, the mistake of eating the apple was severe, but it could have been corrected without major upheaval or expulsion. Man was actually expelled from the Garden for a much more serious error: not for eating the wrong food, but rather for *blaming his wife* (and God)![13] Even so, the Holy One with unconditional Love allowed Adam to return to the Garden briefly, to gather up heavenly spices. These are the gifts that we all need to heal and uplift ourselves on every level, and ultimately to return to the Garden in holiness, with peace of mind, and in perfect health. Later, Adam found a very special cave to bury his wife Chava. We learn that he was initially attracted to this holy place by the Great Light and heavenly fragrance coming from within the cave, and then he realized that this area is one of the entrances to the Garden of Eden. As he chiseled the rock near the opening of the cave, he smelled the sweet fragrance of the Garden, which was familiar to him from the time before he was expelled. He wanted to get closer to the source of this fragrance, and continued to dig until a heavenly voice cried out "Enough! Don't go beyond this point!"[14]

When our forefather Abraham [*Color Plate 9 – The Oak of Abraham*] was chasing a calf that was needed to feed his three angelic guests, he came upon this same cave, known as the "Cave of the Patriarchs" and realized that this was the fitting burial place for his wife Sarah. The first person to rediscover it since Adam, Abraham saw the Great Light there.[15] He also smelled the sweet fragrance that pervaded the cave, the scent of the Garden of Eden, which is identical to the aroma of the Temple Incense.[16] When he began to dig, a heavenly voice proclaimed to him that the first man and his wife were buried there. He then saw them sleeping on two beds, with candles burning over their heads.

According to the Zohar, Abraham's son Isaac [*Color Plate 10 – The Sacrifice of Isaac*] was also mesmerized by the fragrance of this same cave. It says that Isaac saw "two caves that were one" and he went in and saw the *Shechina* (Divine Presence) there. This area is also known as the *Me'arat HaMachpela* (Double Cave) to this day. He then chose a field next to the cave as his regular place for daily prayers. This is the elevated level of prayer that is referred to when we learn that "Isaac went out to pray in the field."[17]

Rabbi Yehuda said "The Holy One made a heavenly Jerusalem above, corresponding to the worldly Jerusalem below." There are seven gates to Jerusalem above, and seven groups of ministering angels that guard them. These are called the Gates of Righteousness and it is through these portals that the souls of the Righteous pass when they leave this world. This holy cave, adjacent to the Garden of Eden, is the first gate that the souls enter. There they are met by Adam, the guardian of that gate. If the soul is worthy, Adam calls out "Make way! May your coming be in Peace!"[18]

This extremely holy cave, which in Judaic tradition is second only to the Temple Mount of Jerusalem in importance, is located in present day Hebron, Israel. This locale has also been known as "*Kiryat Arba*" (City of the Four) since antiquity, because four couples are buried there: Adam and Chava, Abraham and Sarah, Isaac and Rebecca, and Jacob and Leah. Just as Isaac witnessed "two caves that are one" it is called the "Double Cave" because this is the place where heaven and earth meet. The cave illustrates the paradox between that which is holy and sacred compared to that which is coarse and earthly.

This is the one place on earth where the seemingly dual nature of reality can potentially be unified. In the future, the unity of these two realities will be revealed, for what is above is below, and what is below is above.[19] This is the reason why our Sages instituted the phrase *Min HaOlam v'Ad HaOlam* - "from the Upper World to the lower world" - which was said following all Blessings spoken in the Temple, in order to emphasize that the Upper World and lower world are truly one, and that Blessings flow continuously from one to the other.[20]

The Story of Noah[21]

Rabbi Tzadok HaCohen taught that the first time a word or concept appears in the Torah marks its "headquarters" and is the key to knowing and understanding its essence. The second and third times the word comes up are also significant indicators. While this is almost always true, in the case of fragrance, its headquarters in the Torah is actually the place where it is conspicuously **not** mentioned: the Garden of Eden. Paradise was filled with the most beautiful fragrance on earth, yet this is *not mentioned* in the story, nor is anything relating to the sense of smell. As noted previously, this very significant *lack* of any text relating to fragrance indicated to our sages its vital importance.

The first actual mention and therefore the secondary headquarters of fragrance in the Torah occurs in the tale of Noah. After the Flood, Noah came out of the Ark to offer sacrifices. "God smelled the 'appeasing fragrance' - *Rayach Nichoach* (related to the Hebrew name *Noach*) - which brought Him great joy, and God said to Himself, 'Never again will I curse the soil because of man... I will never again strike down all life as I have just done.'"[22] God was very pleased with Noah.

What brought God such great joy? From the Midrash, we learn that before Noah performed the sacrifices, he enrobed himself with the very same aromatic garment which was made from the vestments that God had made for Adam and Eve in the Garden of Eden, and which Noah had brought into the Ark before the Flood. Wearing this mantle, he offered four sacrifices at the future site of the Temple in Jerusalem. We learn that it was actually the fragrance of this holy garment from Eden, more than the aroma of the animal offerings, that God joyfully called an "appeasing fragrance." This inspired Him to make an eternal Rainbow Covenant of protection and guidance for all of humanity.

Towards the very end of the Flood, Noah sent out a dove to see if the water had subsided from the land's surface. It had not. Seven days later, he sent out the dove a second time as "the Gates of the Garden of Eden were opened," and the dove returned with an olive branch. Olive represents a connection to the holy olive oil used in the Menorah, and the aspect of wisdom that closely connects the Menorah with the incense, the fragrance of heaven.

Noah was in the Ark for just over 12 months, from the 17th of Heshvan until the 27th of Heshvan of the following year. His four sacrifices took place the next day, on the 28th. Heshvan is the Hebrew month of darkness, as it is devoid of any holiday until the coming of the Messiah and the future Temple dedication. As we say, throughout time we are on our way from *Mar* ("Bitter") Heshvan to *Ram* ("Exalted") Heshvan. This month is ultimately connected to the Messiah, who will know and judge each person by using his highly refined sense of smell, as it says, the Messiah "*V'Hayrichu et Yirat HaShem* - Smelled the Awe of God."[23] With a highly refined sensitivity to a person's fragrance, the Messiah will know him and what tribe he is from, similar to the way that a master perfumer can precisely identify any given fragrance.

Noah is a universal figure, representing all humanity. The seven Noahide laws are based on the Talmud's teachings regarding ethical behavior for all people and cultures, and were in fact an early source of international law. The Noahide laws relate to justice, blasphemy, idolatry, illicit intercourse, homicide, theft and the humane treatment of animals. The fact that the section regarding Noah is the secondary "headquarters" of aroma in the Torah signifies that the heavenly fragrance and every other aspect of divine revelation is a universal gift given to all nations, and is not limited in any way to the Jewish people and our own traditional practices.

This dispels the myth that God was primarily concerned with His "Chosen People" to the exclusion of all others. Rather, the Jewish people were entrusted with the Noahide laws. It is their mission and responsibility to guard them and teach them to the nations of the world, so that all people everywhere will be imbued with holiness. Aside from the 613 detailed laws of Moses that the Jews were to safeguard and keep exclusively among themselves as an *Am Kadosh* – a Holy People - our ultimate purpose is exercised through keeping and teaching the Noahide laws. We were thus commanded by God at Mt. Sinai, "And you shall be to me a *Mamlechet Cohanim* – a Kingdom of Priests - and a Holy Nation"[24] to teach, bless and safeguard all of humanity, and to be caretakers of all of God's Creation.

According to the classic commentator Sforno, this clearly indicates that the Jewish People are to serve as Priests to all of humanity. Further, he states that in the Messianic Age we will have achieved this goal, as it is written, "You shall be called Priests of the Compassionate One."[25] The primary role of a priest is not to be a "missionary," but rather to serve as a living example of holiness. In this way he will be seen as a messenger of God, and people will be drawn to his teachings. In the words of the Prophet Malachi, "For the lips of the Priest shall safeguard knowledge, and people will seek Torah from his mouth for he is a messenger of the Compassionate One."[26]

Just as people are to seek Torah from the mouth of a Priest, so too will the nations of the earth be drawn to seek Torah from the kingdom of priests when they see that these priests have become a living example of the divine teaching. The people of Israel must therefore strive to become a "Light to the Nations."[27] When we have achieved this goal, we will merit the fulfillment of the prophecy that "Nations will walk in your Light, and sovereigns to the glow of your dawn."[28] The people of Israel were never given an assignment to collectively spread out among the nations and preach the truth of the Torah. Instead, our task is to nurture the seed of the divine teaching within us. In this way, we can become an ethical and spiritual model that will inspire all people to accept the universal principles of the Torah, and in particular the seven Noahide laws.

The Blessings of Isaac[29]

The second mention of aroma in the Torah occurs when Isaac gave his blessings to Jacob, who was wearing the same aromatic garment of Noah, preserved from the Garden of Eden. Wearing this special mantle, which their mother Rifka had obtained from Esav, Jacob entered the room where Isaac was resting. He brought with him the fragrance of the Garden of Eden,[30] along with the food for his father that his mother had prepared. It was God's plan that Isaac would not recognize Jacob visually or by touch. He ate and drank. He then asked his son to kiss him in order to establish a close contact, so that Jacob would merit his blessing. With that kiss, Isaac inhaled the heavenly scent filling the air, the Holy Spirit rested upon him, and he suddenly realized that the one who wore that garment must be a righteous person, the one worthy of his blessing.

"[Jacob] approached [the bed] and kissed him. [Isaac] smelled the fragrance of his garment and blessed him. See, my son's fragrance is like the perfume of a field blessed by God."[31] Isaac smelled the fragrance of paradise on Jacob's garment, and remembered the *Rayach haSadeh* - "Fragrance of the Field," the heavenly smell of the Garden of Eden. He had experienced it before when he was bound by his father Abraham to be sacrificed on Mt. Moriah,[32] and also he had generated this scent in his prayers. This happened when he was standing in a field by the Cave of the Patriarchs, praying for his children. When his future wife Rebecca rode up on her camel, a divine fragrance came forth that was familiar to Isaac, and he was suddenly reminded of his previous unforgettable ecstatic experience. The Zohar explains that when the Torah relates that Isaac went out to pray in the field, he "saw two caves that are one," and when he went inside the cave, he saw the Divine Presence, and smelled the heavenly fragrance of the Garden of Eden. He then made this special location his regular place of prayer.

This headquarters of aroma in the Torah illustrates that a righteous person, through the power of deep prayer and meditation, can emanate the fragrance of the Temple incense and the Garden of Eden. Isaac prayed to find his soulmate, and that they would have children who would be worthy descendants of his father Abraham. Later, when Isaac smelled Jacob approach him with a tasty meal, his Holy Spirit was activated, and he realized that the person standing before him must be the answer to his prayers. He foresaw that his descendents would build the Temple on Mt. Moriah, and offer sacrifices in Jerusalem. Isaac then gave Jacob ten blessings, corresponding to the ten "Pronouncements" with which God created the world, indicating that in the merit of this son, the world would continue to exist.

In this particular episode in the Torah, our Rabbis teach us that there is a play on the closely linked words *beged* – garment, and *boged* – traitors, which have only slightly different vowels. We learn from this that even the souls that dwell in the most evil people will ultimately be repaired, returned to God, and give forth the beautiful fragrance of the Garden of Eden. That deep realization came to Isaac, who was blind, when he smelled the heavenly fragrance of Jacob's garment. He saw prophetically that the most broken places in people's lives, including his own, will ultimately be fixed. Thus, Isaac foresaw that people will depart from God throughout time, but will also have the potential to return to Him in complete Holiness. The garment had a most divine fragrance when Jacob wore it.[33]

The Story of Joseph[34]

According to the Me'am Loez, the special "coat of many colors" that Jacob gave to his son Joseph was the same aromatic garment that was passed down to him from the Garden of Eden. This "rainbow coat" is the vestment which aroused so much jealousy among Joseph's brothers that they dipped a fragment of it in blood, and presented this as evidence to Jacob that Joseph had been killed by a wild beast.

Joseph's brothers sold him to a caravan of Ishmaelite spice traders who were on their way to Egypt, and he was transported with a shipment of gum, resin and balsam (the chief Temple incense spice). The only other time when these three aromatic materials are mentioned together in the Torah is when Jacob instructs his sons to bring the Egyptian viceroy (secretly Joseph) a gift of "a little balsam and honey, some gum and resin...." Throughout their journey, the brothers were surrounded by these fragrances.

The reason that these spices were prophetically chosen relates to the peculiar properties of aroma, since the sense of smell has the capacity to take one back through a vast span of time and trigger vivid memories. Memories of significant past events, and even memories of experiences from former lifetimes can be awakened by certain fragrances, such as Lot - labdanum, which is one of the gifts that Jacob instructed his sons to bring to Egypt. The moment when the brothers, initially identified as righteous men by the Torah, were propelled towards complete repentance was marked by their adamant refusal to allow Benjamin to suffer the same fate as Joseph by being incarcerated in Pharaoh's prison. Divine Providence stepped in. While they waited to meet with Joseph, it is conceivable that the brothers were transported back to the time when they sold Joseph, partly influenced by the aroma of the spice gifts they carried.

This set the stage for the dramatic reconciliation with their long-lost brother. Similarly, the Torah emphasizes that aromatic sacrifices, and in particular the Temple incense, aim to transport God Himself back to the time before the First Sin, as it were, to a time of perfection in Paradise. This is perhaps why God tells us that the Temple incense brings Him exalted joy. The fragrance of the incense also had an incredibly elevating effect on the mentality of all people who experienced it, awakening their very highest consciousness level, known as *Nevuah* - Prophecy.

The idea of being transported back to a time before iniquity was in the world is epitomized by the Incense. Balsam and Labdanum evoke a memory of the sin of the sale of Joseph, and the atonement for it. Further, the foul-smelling galbanum in the incense mixture eternally reminds us, in aromatic form, of our past mistakes. Despite its rank odor, rather than repel, it mysteriously binds together with the ten other sweet smelling spices in perfect aromatic harmony.[35]

Moses: Receiving the Torah[36]

According to the famous Kabbalist Rabbi Yitzhak Luria, the first man and Moses were both *Neshamot Klaliot* – "general souls," who contained sparks of all the souls in the world. Thus their lives are a vital teaching, and have relevance, to all people for all time.

The exact recipes for both the Temple incense and the holy anointing oil were revealed to Moses during the transmission of the Torah that he received on Mt. Sinai after the Exodus. This included the precise ingredients, proportions, other materials needed, secret methods of preparation and use, as well as the procedure for burning the incense on the "*Mizbayach Zahav*" - the "golden incense altar."[37] Although no animals were sacrificed on the incense altar, it was called a *Mizbayach* – "slaughtering place," because the incense had the power to break, subjugate and slaughter evil. The anointing oil and incense are deeply connected, and each of them is considered to be *Kodesh Kadoshim* - Holiest of the Holy.

The Talmud teaches us that when Moses ascended to the top of Mt. Sinai to receive the Torah, "As each of the ten Commandments was spoken by the Holy One, Blessed be He, the world was filled with fragrance."[38] This refers to the fragrance of paradise, which is the scent of the Temple incense. As a special gift, Moses was taught an important secret about the Temple incense by the Angel of Death. It was revealed to him that the incense has the power of life (and power over death), and could be used to stop a deadly plague. When Moses ascended to the most heavenly place on Mt. Sinai, the angels were opposed to giving the Torah to mankind. They wanted the divine revelation to remain in heaven.

God: "Moses, you have to give them an answer."

Moses: "But they will burn me with the fire of their breath!"

God: "Hold on to my Throne of Glory from which I have carved out the souls of the People of Israel, and then you will be able to answer the angels."

In other words, Moses was instructed to hang on to the souls of the 600,000 people of Israel. From their strength, he would be able to give the angels an answer, and by being connected to these souls, which are eternal, he would not be harmed by the fire of the angels' breath. The souls of Israel are stronger than the angels, and Moses will be on the level of eternity and able to rule over them. Even though God had already determined that we would receive the Torah, Moses had to lay out the claim for his people and mankind before the angels, who were previously bound into partnership with God in the creation of man.

When Moses passionately explained that we humans truly need the Torah to guide us to live lives of holiness in spite of all of the challenges and difficulties we face, all of the angels were deeply moved, and fell in love with him. It is written, "You went on High, you captured the hearts of the angels, and they gave you Gifts."[39] Each angel gave Moses a gift of knowledge which was of crucial importance, and supplemented the Torah knowledge that was given to him directly by God.

Even the Angel of Death, who was originally opposed to man's creation, gave Moses a special gift: the amazing secret that the Temple incense has the power of life over death. While all of the other details regarding the incense were revealed directly to Moses by God, this secret, which would soon save the Jewish people from extinction, was exclusively in this angel's domain, and thus could only be revealed according to his will: "If the Angel of Death had not taught Moses (that only the Temple incense has the power to overcome death), how else could he have known?"[40]

Because of this gift, Moses had the crucial knowledge to order Aaron to walk through the camp with the burning incense when the plague of death broke out in the wilderness, since he knew that the 11 Ketoret spices have the power to fully overcome death and evil. Although this life-saving use of the incense was permitted only as a one-time event, we learn from this episode that in a time of plague, there is no remedy better than the incense. "Aaron took the incense pan, as Moses had commanded him. He offered it to atone for the people. He was standing between the dead and the living (with the burning incense), and the plague was stopped."[41] At first the plague was checked, and Aaron was able to save the lives of the remaining people, and bring all of the ill back to good health. Then the plague was completely nullified, and even the people who had died came back to life again! Aaron bound up the Angel of Death so he could not rule over them at that moment, totally taking away his destroying power.

This is evidence that the Temple incense can stop a plague. Remarkably, merely reciting with deep concentration the mystical words of the incense verses - *Pitum HaKetoret* - also has this same power. This reading, which is included in Chapter 3, is permitted to anyone at any time, and this is the secret of the key words *Kach lecha Samim* ("take unto yourself spices"): For your pleasure, for your health, to eliminate impurities, and to save your life.

The Temple Mount

The original fragrant sacrifices took place at Mount Moriah, the future location of the Temple and the Holy of Holies in Jerusalem [*Color Plate 11 – Jerusalem*]: Adam was created from the dust of Mt. Moriah. Shortly after he was expelled from the Garden of Eden he built an altar, and offered the original incense sacrifice. On the first anniversary of the world's creation, Cain and Abel brought sacrifices on the altar that was built by Adam. Noah built his altar at this same location, and made his four sacrifices there right after leaving the Ark. Abraham brought Isaac to sacrifice him at this same place. Isaac was praying at this very location when a caravan of camels arrived with his future wife. Many authorities state that this was also the spot where Jacob had his famous dream of a ladder rising to heaven, with angels ascending and descending. Jacob called this place "God's Temple" and "The Gate to Heaven."[42] According to the Midrash, Jacob's dream was an allusion to the future Temple service, and the angels represent High Priests sending fragrant offerings up to heaven.

We thus learn that the Temple Mount is the geographical headquarters of fragrance on the planet, and it is also the setting for the story of Creation. The two are deeply linked. Further, we learn that "the gate of the Garden of Eden is very close to the Temple Mount." From the fact that the headquarters of fragrance and of creation are the same in the Torah, we derive that the fragrance of the Garden of Eden (Paradise) is identical with that of the Temple incense.[43]

Another concept about the location of the creation story is that it is "not of this world," that is, not a geographical location in this world *as we know it*. These two concepts are reconciled by a Midrash which says, "Adam was created from the earth of the place of his Atonement." Both Adam's creation and his sacrifices occurred at the Temple Mount, a special high-energy place on the planet, which is actually a "portal to another world" in much the same way that a woman's womb is a portal to another world.

The offering required of Abraham, the sacrifice of his own son, was different from all of the other offerings brought on the Temple Mount. Our sages declare that this was our Patriarch's most important journey. Abraham demonstrated to the entire world the extent that one must go to in order to prove faithfulness and show honor to the Holy One. In reaching such a high level, Abraham and Isaac beheld a vision of the Temple that would stand at that same location in the future, and Abraham declared that the Temple should one day be built at that very location on Mt. Moriah. The Temple thus represents the pinnacle of self-sacrifice and devotion to the Holy One, an essential level of moral and spiritual purification that will set the stage for the redemption of the world and the arrival of the Messiah.

Most significant is that we can actually **do something** to comfort the "Divine sense of smell" because the Temple incense sacrifice produces an appeasing and joyful fragrance to God. This offering brings immense joy and satisfaction to the Creator, appeasing His anger and drawing down life and blessings to His creation. This first happened on the 28th of Heshvan when Noah offered his sacrifices. The completion of the Solomon's Temple also happened in Heshvan, the month related to "fixing our sense of smell." The Sanctuary wandered from Mt. Sinai from place to place for 440 years. Finally, King David [*Color Plate 12 – The Youth David*] brought the Ark up to Jerusalem, and built an Altar on Mt. Moriah. His son Solomon completed the work, and at the dedication ceremony declared that the Holy Temple was to be a House of Prayer for the people of Israel, and for all people on earth. Visitors would be moved by the breathtaking outer beauty, as well as the extraordinary inner, spiritual manifestation of the awesome Divine Presence [*Color Plate 13 – Jerusalem Pilgrimage*].

Today, while we have no Temple, the sacrifices have been replaced by our prayers, including the recital of the verses describing the incense offering. The best preparation for this is by purifying ourselves, by seeking the very greatest level of health for our body, and the highest level of consciousness. As a result, if we seek to attain optimum health and purity, the body becomes a "Temple" and begins to emanate a fragrance similar to the Temple incense and the Garden of Eden. By doing so we bring joy to our Creator; our sincere efforts in this regard are considered in heaven to be just as worthy today as the incense offering was and will be in the days of the Temple.

The Temple and Jerusalem

When Adam was expelled from the Garden of Eden, he was returned to Mt. Moriah where he had previously been created "from the dust."[44] He would remain there to serve God until the day of his death. On that day, man stood there on the Temple Mount and cried before the Angels, and out of deep compassion, they offered to do whatever he wanted. Adam requested of the Angels that he be permitted to bring spices out of the Garden along with him, saying: "Just let me take along some of these sweet smelling things from the Garden, the pleasant fragrances, and I will make a sacrifice offering to God so He will answer me, *and then I can ultimately return.*" The Holy One agreed, and the Angels temporarily let Adam back into the Garden, so that he could take seeds for food, fragrant plants, and aromatic spices, including the spices of the Temple incense.[45] Adam represents collective humanity for all time, and to this day, the angels are still assisting in this process, overseeing the healing powers of the medicinal plants. These crucial botanicals were always intended to fully restore our body and soul, so we can return to the Garden in our original state of perfect wellbeing.

One mystical text mentions four of the eleven Ketoret spices that Adam took from the Garden: frankincense, galbanum, balsam and spikenard. On that first day of his exile from the Garden, with these spices, man produced and burned the very first Temple incense offering on the Temple Mount, the most natural place on earth for fragrance to bring atonement.[46] Another source confirms that the spices of the Temple incense were taken from the Garden of Eden.[47] We deduce from this that the incense had the very same fragrance as the Garden of Eden, because our sources state that from the aroma of his offering, Adam remembered his former home in Paradise. This is the first instance of **memory** that ever occurred, according to our holy tradition. That is why **fragrance imprints on memory** and is so deeply connected with it, and also why our primordial ancient collective memory is actually all about fragrance and the Garden of Eden.

When we remember the time and place "before the Original Sin," we are reaching back to a powerful ancient memory of fragrances and spices in the Garden. It has so far remained only a memory, as we learn that no one will be permitted to fully return to that holy place until the time of the Messiah. Then we will finally collectively make the repair of all of the repercussions of the First Sin, and make our return. Yet according to our holy tradition, this is why natural fragrances can evoke such powerful healing: *they bring back the ancient memory of Paradise.* Thus when we often say "until the time of the Messiah ('Anointed one')" it could also be interpreted to mean, "until the time when a person is anointed (with fragrant oils)."

There is a classic story from an early Midrash about two brothers who lived in adjacent valleys in ancient Israel where they shared agricultural land, divided by a mountain ridge. One brother was married and had many children, while the other brother lived alone. One day, after they harvested their wheat together, they divided the grain equally between them and each took home five full bushel baskets. That night, neither brother could sleep. The bachelor brother decided that his brother needed and deserved the larger share of the wheat to feed his big family, so in the middle of the night he took one of his baskets of wheat, carried it over the mountain ridge and secretly left it at his brother's home together with his brother's five wheat baskets.

Meanwhile that same night, the married brother was unable to sleep, thinking that his single brother would need more wealth to take a bride, and build his home and family. So he also secretly climbed the ridge, and transferred a basket of wheat to his brother's storehouse. In the morning, when both brothers awoke, each discovered that, to his utter amazement, he still had five baskets of wheat! Each thought that the Holy One had brought about a great miracle as a reward for his kind deed. The story was repeated a few months later when they harvested figs. Each secretly transferred twice the amount of figs to the other brother in the middle of the night, and then awoke in the morning to discover that his own supply was still miraculously undiminished.

Finally the time of the grape harvest arrived, and again the brothers harvested together and divided their produce equally. This time each brother decided to deliver his *entire share* of the harvest to his brother, who really deserved it. As fate would have it, the brothers bumped into each other at the top of the ridge in the dead of night. Suddenly they both realized what had been happening all along. They embraced, danced together and wept with tears of joy.

This event fixed the great tragedy of Cain and Abel.[48] Cain had the idea to make an offering to the Holy One, and then Abel improved on it. Abel's offering was accepted, but Cain's was not, which caused Cain to become angry, depressed, and jealous of his brother. Cain killed his brother in a fit of anger, but since nobody had ever died before, he did not fully realize what he was doing. Abel should have tried to teach his brother how to offer a sacrifice properly, and Cain should have respected his brother instead of lashing out at him in revenge. From the day this tragedy was fixed until today, this ridge has been known as Mt. Moriah (*Moriya* in Hebrew means the "Myrrh of God"). Myrrh "tears" came to be known as one of the most important of all spices, and at this location, the Temple incense - containing resinous "tears" of myrrh, frankincense, costus and galbanum - was offered especially to bring great tears of joy to God.

Jerusalem was always the focal point of the Holy Land of Israel, and the *Bet HaMikdash* – the Temple, which stood on the top of Mt. Moriah, is the focal point of Jerusalem. The breathtakingly magnificent First Temple, once called one of the "Seven Wonders of the World," was built by King Solomon and stood for 410 years before it was ruthlessly destroyed by the Babylonians. After a seventy year exile, a small group of Jews returned to Jerusalem from Babylon and constructed the Second Temple, which stood for 420 years before its destruction by the Roman legions in 70 AD. The Second Temple was said to be a poor rendition, smaller in stature and lacking most of the original Holy Vessels (including the Ark of the Covenant) which made Solomon's Temple far more majestic. Of this mere shadow of former glory it was disparagingly said, "This House is nothing!"

The vital task of building the Temple could not be accomplished until the Israelites had settled in the Promised Land, appointed a King, and attained peace with the surrounding nations. The Torah then continues, "When you cross the Jordan, dwelling in the Land which the Lord your God gives you to inherit, and He gives you rest from all your enemies round about so that you dwell in safety; then there shall be the place which the Lord your God will choose, to make His Name dwell there."[49] These conditions were finally attained during the days of Solomon. The services in the Temple were a complete reversal of the forces of creation, when God transformed the spiritual elements into physical form; here, the physical elements of existence were completely uplifted and imbued with spirituality.

One of the 613 commandments of the Torah that is incumbent upon the Jewish people is to build the Temple, as it says, "You shall seek [God's] habitation."[50] Thus in each generation in which the Holy Temple is not rebuilt, it is as if it has been destroyed. Since the Second Temple was conquered and destroyed due to *sinat hinam* - needless, reckless hatred - it can only be rebuilt through *ahavat hinam* - unconditional love. This requires that the Jewish leadership take an active role in greatly emphasizing what unites the Jewish people, and not what divides them.

The essence of the Temple is the indwelling of the *Shechina* - Divine Presence - in the heart of every Jewish person (and by extension, in the hearts of all humanity). If the people of Israel sanctify themselves by performing the 613 commandments of the Torah, all of which are rooted above, then God will not only dwell in the Temple, but most importantly, God will dwell in the **heart of each person** as it is written, "They shall make for Me a Temple, and I will dwell *within them*."[51] Thus, when Israel destroyed the "Inner Temple" of the heart through needless hatred, the external facade of the building was no longer of any use, and so it was also destroyed and abandoned.[52]

In the Temple, an animal was sacrificed to atone for (and to replace on the Altar) the person bringing a sin offering. The headquarters of this in the Torah is when Abraham attempts to sacrifice Isaac, but God replaces him with a ram. Abraham set this process in motion with this sacrifice, and by saying the morning prayer, which builds a vision of perfection; each blessing voices the prayer of a different part of the body. The light of the mind, in full consciousness, is like the fire of the incense altar that unlocks the fragrant perfume of devotion through the body, from deep within the Soul.

We reached this level as a nation when we built the desert *Mishkan*

– Tabernacle - *exactly* the way that God directed us to, even though most of us were unskilled and unprepared for this task [*Plates 17 and 18 – Desert Tabernacle and Tabernacle at Gilgal, courtesy of Vendyl Jones*]. God instructed us at Mt. Sinai, "They shall make for Me a Sanctuary [the Tabernacle], and I will dwell inside them."[53] God proclaimed that He would dwell within the heart of each and every person. A remarkable portable structure (about 20 feet high, 24 feet wide, and 64 feet long), the Tabernacle could be taken apart and transported from place to place as it accompanied us through our desert journey. It was meant to be a microcosm of the entire creation, teaching man that he has the responsibility to elevate and sanctify every aspect of his life. It represented man's partnership with God in bringing all of creation to its final culmination. Thus, building the Tabernacle was man's way of replicating God's act of creating the entire universe.

After all the components were ready, the Tabernacle had to be completely set up by Moses, but then taken down again each day for the first seven days. Moses did not lose patience, and he finally got everything set up perfectly. Our Rabbis teach that even when he set it up correctly, it still had to be taken down, to teach us to not be attached to results. We are a work in progress, and just doing the process with the right intention brings us closer to God – even if we do not necessarily achieve the "final goal." Every person in this world has something to repair, or he wouldn't be here. Mainly we are here to fix ourselves, but also to interact with others, which forces us to do additional or intensified repair work. It is not perfection (which would take us out of this world), but the continual striving for perfection that is the key.

The Power of Prayer

We have learned that a righteous person, through the power of deep prayer and meditation, can begin to emanate the fragrance of the Temple incense and the Garden of Eden. According to our teachers, holy prayer is a perfect integration of body and soul. One of the goals of prayer is to align our personal will with God's Divine Will, which is possible when all blockages are removed and we are brought to a state of harmony. The first step on the path of intense devotional prayer is to attach the root level of our soul to the Light of the Creator. This is done by special preparation involving washing, anointment and meditation. One then proceeds to draw down the Light of God, the vital force which permeates every cell of his body, into all of his being. In this way, all the limbs of his body become elevated, and included in the *kavanna* – intention - of prayer. When cleaned of all impurity, our body becomes a Temple for our soul. This is what is meant by "direct your heart to the Holy Temple" and this is how God can dwell within us.

Just like physical coupling, prayer must take place in a state of arousal, passion, and joy if it is to bear fruit, and passion requires full involvement of the body – you can't just be "Spirit," leave your body, and start praying. Draw the energy into the temple of your body, and from that place allow yourself to become spiritually aroused so your prayers will bear fruit. The body is the fuel for the soul's fire. We allow our bodies to be "dissolved" into our souls and the light surrounding the body. Then through our prayer consciousness we emit a beautiful scent, corresponding to the *Rayach Nichoach* - sweet fragrance - of the Temple Incense.[54]

Since we currently do not have the Temple, it is all the more important for us to re-enact the Temple sacrifices on a personal level. On the larger community level we do this with a *Minyan* - a quorum of ten men or ten women. We offer up our pure intention in prayer, which is returned to us and our purified personal Temple as the gift of life. In this way we acknowledge God's presence in the world. The fragrance we emit each moment is a perfect reflection of the physical, emotional and spiritual chemistry that is happening inside of us.

On the deepest level, a pathway has been identified by our sages and mystics that allows us to seek guidance from the Holy One, even in the midst of confusion, when every step forward raises questions and concern. Rabbi Nachman of Breslov, among others, taught that *Hisboddedus* is the practice of frequently and regularly speaking to God, privately and in a very personal way. We communicate in our mother tongue, speaking with the Holy One as our closest friend and partner in life. This approach is even deeper than our set prayers, and allows us to go into a very profound conversation and relationship with the Great Spirit.

Chapter 3

Incense: the Sacred Fragrance of the Temple

The Hebrew word ***Ketoret*** – incense - is from the root word **KaTaR** which means "steam" or "smoke." Resh Lakish teaches that this root word refers to smoke that produces a fragrance, which elevates us to a higher place. The Jerusalem Temple incense takes us to lofty heights just as an animal sacrifice brings us to a higher level. In every way, the incense sacrifice is sent straight up to heaven, as a pleasant fragrance to the Holy One as it also elevates the people of Israel.

Each day, the High Priest's morning began (and afternoon ended) with Holy ***KeToReT***. From the Midrash Tanchuma we learn that the word Ketoret is an acronym of four elements: ***K****edusha* - Holiness, embracing our sacred mission; ***T****ahara* - Purity, to cleanse the spirit; ***Ra****chamim* – Mercy, generosity; and ***T****ikva* - Hope, replacing despair with the vision of a bright future. The incense is meant to light up our darkest places, unite our bodies and souls in the service of God, and imbue our lives with holiness, purity, compassion and hope. The aroma of the incense recalls the essence of the Garden of Eden *before* the creation of man, when it was completely pure and without any sin. As it says in our holy teachings, "The aroma of the Temple incense is a true reminder of the fragrance of the Garden of Eden."[1]

On Mt. Sinai, Moses was commanded to build a *Mishkan* - portable desert Tabernacle - to allow God's presence to dwell among the people. The Holy One instructed him how to build this portable Temple in every detail. Even though most of us were unskilled as master craftsmen, we constructed everything perfectly, taking the spiritual dimension and artistically manifesting it as a physical reality. Including all of the elements of the Jerusalem Temple, yet much less elaborate, the Tabernacle is a divine model of how the world should be, representing all of creation - a perfect microcosm of our relationship with God. The portability of the Tabernacle demonstrated that our relationship with God is not dependent on *where* we are. When we finally arrived in Israel and built the Temple in Jerusalem, the Ark of the Covenant that we constructed and carried through the desert as the centerpiece of the Tabernacle was placed in the most sacred area, known as the Holy of Holies.

In the Torah, the Temple incense is mentioned immediately after the mention of Aaron and his descendants, known as the *Cohanim* – the priests, linking the two eternally together.[2] Although the incense offering was performed only by the Priests, as a special one-time exception, the very first offerings in the Tabernacle were performed by Aaron's brother Moses, a Levite. This special exception had to be made, as Aaron and his sons were still in the process of being initiated, and so could not yet make the offerings themselves. This initiation period was a special consecration of the entire Mishkan/Offering/Temple Service process, from HaShem to Moses, and from Moses to Aaron and his sons. It was not only an initiation for the priests, but for all of Israel, establishing a bridge between heaven and earth. All future Temple services and all future actions on our part meant to invoke the offerings of the Temple service are thus re-enactments, acts of confirmation, of what happened during those first days of the Tabernacle in the wilderness many years ago.[3]

These initial offerings took place during the seven day inauguration period of the *Mishkan*, about six months after construction began. Each of those seven days, Moses set up the Tabernacle and then took it down again. At that time he served in the role of a priest, wearing a white hemless garment as the priests did, offering the incense on a golden altar and transcending time. Finally, on the eighth day, which was *Rosh Hodesh* - the first day of the Hebrew month of *Nisan*, Moses set up the Tabernacle perfectly and let it remain up. Aaron offered the Temple incense on that day, and this awesome honor and responsibility remained in the hands of his priestly family forever after. This date on our calendar thus marks the New Year for the Temple incense, and also the New Year for Kings and Months.

On that first day, and during the following eleven days, each of the heads of the twelve tribes consecutively donated incense for use on the outer altar. Each day a different *Nasi* donated, in the order designated on Mt. Sinai. "One golden incense bowl weighing ten (shekels) filled with Temple incense" was brought as a private gift during these days when the *Mishkan* was first dedicated.[4] The first prince to make this donation was Nachshon ben Aminadav of the tribe of Yehuda, who was the first person to bravely enter into the Red Sea, and one of the only men to complete the entire journey from Egypt and enter the land of Israel. This very first incense offering was conducted by Moses on the main *outer* altar, which was to be used thereafter only for the animal sacrifices.[5] This dedication period was a special twelve day event, and forever after the Incense would always be donated (in effect) by the entire congregation, and never by a single individual.[6] After this celebration period, the incense would be offered only on the *inner* golden incense altar inside the *Kodesh* – the Holy Place, within the Tabernacle or Temple.

It is interesting that Nachshon was the first to make a donation, because the root of his name is *nachash* - snake, the ancient symbol in the Near East for the secret mystic orders. This word is also the root of *nachoshet* – copper, which is mentioned many times as a building material for the Tabernacle. In the Hebrew mystical tradition, copper is the metal that corresponds to fire, whereas the metal which corresponds to air is gold. It seems very fitting that it is Nachshon, the "copper snake," and the element of fire, who donates the inaugural incense offering for the altar covered in gold, the air element. Where is water? It is in the person of Moses, who actually performs the initial Temple incense offering, made from the produce of the earth.[3]

During the days of the Tabernacle, and for over 800 years during the First and Second Temples, about 2.5 lbs of Temple incense were ignited every evening, and the same amount was burned again in the morning.[7] Another opinion states that only about 0.5 lb was offered each time. The incense ceremony was performed by a specially-chosen priest as a once-in-a-lifetime opportunity. It was a great *segula* - divine Blessing - to offer the incense, and it is said that a priest who did so would be greatly blessed in all areas of his life, including very good *parnassa* - financial livelihood. The one who offered would become wealthy, have a long life and continual divine protection.

Before the third *Payis* – the Temple lottery, which determined who would offer the incense that day, a priest proclaimed in the courtyard of the Temple, "New priests! (those who had never offered incense before) Come and draw lots for the incense!"[8] There were always enough new priests available to hold a lottery, and there were two such lotteries per day, one for each incense offering.

The Temple incense works on the very highest consciousness level. Since the soul, mind and physical body are all deeply connected, *all levels* of a person's being are ultimately affected in the most beneficial way by being brought to a state of abundant life and vibrant health. Women throughout the Jerusalem area did not commonly wear perfume during the Temple days; even a bride was not required to perfume herself, because everyone preferred to experience the holy fragrance which emanated from the incense. The Talmud relates that the Ketoret fragrance reached as far away as Jericho (about 20 miles from Jerusalem, and 3,000 feet *lower* in elevation), and goats in Jericho would sneeze from the piquant aroma in the air. This is in spite of the fact that the smoke of the incense always rose straight upwards.

Much greater than that, the ever-present fragrance of the Temple incense brought an extremely elevated level of consciousness to all the people who experienced it. During Temple days, due to the enlightening fragrance in the air, at one time there were *over one million people* in the Jerusalem area on the very lofty spiritual level called Nevuah - Prophecy. The Talmud states, "Many Prophets arose in Israel, double the number of adult males that departed from Egypt."[9] Still, as great as it was having the Prophets in our midst, and as awesome as it was having the Temple with the service of the priests and the incense, it was foreseen that this could only be a temporary taste of something that would eventually be given to all of mankind. This is hinted at in the Midrash: "The Holy One declared, 'In this world, only selected individuals became Prophets, but in the future world, all of Israel will attain full Prophecy.'"[10]

Even when prophecy is truly from God, the person's ability to properly receive, translate and articulate the prophecy depends on that person's spiritual development, and on the training and discipline he has received in the mystic arts. Once achieved, the level of prophecy further depends upon a person's purified state of mind/body/soul and his ability to hear, receive and translate accurately what he encounters. The fragrance of the Temple incense, combined with the holiness of being in Israel, and following God's commandments, all helped to create a state of mind conducive to prophecy. Schools of Prophecy arose with as many as tens of thousands of students at any given time.[3]

The incense service represents the unity of Israel, partly because the eleven spices that make up the incense represent all different types of people. According to the Zohar, the Temple incense offering was the most beloved of all the sacrifices in the eyes of God. The other Sacrifices were brought to express thanks or to make atonement for some sin. The incense however had no "ulterior motive" - its sole purpose was to bring joy to the Holy One. As a byproduct of this Divine Joy above, those who experienced the incense below were elevated to the very highest level of consciousness. In this respect, the Temple incense offering is much greater than prayer: Prayer was instituted as a substitute for the sacrifices, but the incense was far more important to God, on a higher level than any of the other offerings. As proof, we see that the altar for animal and other sacrifices stood outside the Tabernacle, before the entrance. The Temple incense altar was in a much more sacred area, inside the Holy Place next to the Golden Menorah, separated only by a curtain from the divine Ark of the Covenant.

It is written, "Oil and incense make the heart rejoice."[11] Both of these articles and their sacred use bring joy to the Holy One. Thus the Anointing oil and the Temple incense were ordained by God only to make His Heart rejoice, and God is the heart of the universe. As above, so below, and thus all of our hearts are also uplifted. This is also why the Menorah and Temple incense were so closely bound together: "At the time when the Menorah was lit, the Incense was burned."[12]

Aaron and the specially chosen priests who followed in his ways would first prepare and light the wicks of the golden Menorah, and then ignite the incense on the golden altar. The Menorah, the vessel for light, always represents *chochma* – Wisdom - and higher consciousness. This light connects directly to the Temple incense, which is the universal healing medicine. Many believe that the Menorah is based on the shape and appearance of the Moriah plant of Israel. The Menorah has seven arms, three on each side of a central stem. This is the three pronged Hebrew letter *Shin* of this world on one side, and the four pronged *Shin* of the "World to Come" on the other, including the central arm. So the Menorah is the unification of heaven and earth, of this world and the next, of white fire and black fire. The incense produces smoke that contains both black and white smoke within it, and this may also represent the black and white fire of the Hebrew letters inscribed upon the Torah scroll. This includes the Torah that was scribed by the Hand of God, given with the first set of tablets, as well as the second tablets, crafted by Moses.[3]

The fragrance of the incense purified people from sin, as whoever smelled this aroma would have thoughts of repentance. His heart would be purified from all evil thinking, and from the defilement of the evil inclination. No one else was permitted inside the Holies when a priest ignited the incense. Offered in a secret and private way, it makes atonement for *Lashon Hara* - evil speech, which is also said in private, breaking the power of the "Other Side," so he could speak no evil.

"God said to Moses: Take fragrances of balsam, tziporren, galbanum and pure frankincense, all of the same weight - *bod vebod yehiye* - of equal measure, and mixed together simultaneously - as well as (seven other specified) fragrances. Make (the mixture) into incense, as compounded by a master perfumer, well-blended, pure and holy. Grind it very finely, and place it before the (Ark of) Testimony in the Communion Tent where I commune with you. It shall be a Holy of Holies to you. Do not duplicate the formula of the incense that you are making for personal use, since it must remain sacred to God. If a person makes it to enjoy its fragrance, he shall be cut off (spiritually) from his people."[13]

The names of all eleven spices of the Temple Incense are enumerated in the Talmud,[14] and are repeated daily in the morning service. The names and proportions are:

Balsam (chief spice): *70 manot* - measures

Galbanum (vile resin): *70 manot*

Tziporren (clove or shell?): *70 manot*

Frankincense (resin): *70 manot*

Myrrh (resin): *16 manot*

Spikenard (root): *16 manot*

Saffron (flower tops): *16 manot*

Cassia (Chinese cinnamon bark): *16 manot*

Costus (resin): *12 manot*

Cinnamon (bark): *3 manot*

Cinnamon (leaf): *9 manot*

The total of 368 measures is enough for one portion (the amount needed for two incense offerings) for each day of the year, and three additional measures for Yom Kippur. "Make the mixture into incense as compounded by a master perfumer, well blended, pure and holy."[15] Here we see that it is a positive commandment in the Torah to make the incense correctly. The Torah specifies that it should be made in the same manner as the best perfumers produce the finest incenses. Each material had to be cleaned, then ground very finely, mixed together well, and the incense made with absolute purity in every respect. The Torah also specifies that the incense must be holy. This means that the tools, ingredients and labor must be purchased with consecrated money. If anything was unclean, or if it was not purchased with consecrated money, the final product could not be used in the Temple.

The four primary spices in the group of eleven, those that were 70 measures each, together made up nearly 80% of the incense mixture. Balsam, *tzipporen* (exact identity unknown), galbanum and frankincense each comprised 19.8% of the mixture, and only these four major spices are specifically named in the written Torah: "*nataf u'shechelet ve'chelbena...ulevonah zakah.*" Naming them in this way can be seen to imply a real-life process of unfolding creation from potential to actuality. These four major spices represent four stages of the creation of the material world, including both the actual ingredients of the incense, as well as the more abstract levels of astrophysical, cosmological, and spiritual realities of life, as follows:

Nataf is Judaic **Balsam**: Creation begins with a single drop or ball of energy, smaller than the size of an atom, containing everything in the universe in a state of extreme heat beyond our comprehension. This ball of energy explodes and gives birth to space, time, and all energy and matter. ***Shechelet*** is ***Tzipporen***: The physical universe then begins to inflate and expand, although it is still much too hot for matter to appear. ***Chelbena*** is **Galbanum**: Planet Earth cools down enough under the proper conditions to support life, and human history begins. Israel receives the Torah on Sinai and Moses descends, his face shining with the glow of heavenly light. Israel is given the mission to transform matter into Spirit, emulating the way that God transformed Spirit into matter. Moses builds the Tabernacle, and later Solomon builds the first Temple in Jerusalem, where Heaven kisses Earth in the Holy of Holies between the cherubim. ***Levonah*** *zakah* is pure **Frankincense**: Now our mission is to recognize the inner holiness in everything, and prepare the world to receive the ultimate radiance of Godliness, which will completely transform reality on planet Earth back into an eternal Garden of Eden.[16]

Judaic **Balsam** (*Commiphora opobalsamum*) is the chief spice of the Temple incense, and it is in the same botanical family as myrrh. This material was also processed into an anointing oil known as *Shemen Afarsimon*, used as a substitute for the anointing oil of Moses, after King Josiah hid the original oil away just before the destruction of the First Temple. It is mentioned in the Bible by various names, including *Afarsimon, Besem, Bosem, Kataf, Nataf,* and *Tzori*. Balsam is a thorny shrub that stands 10 to 12 feet high, with wand-like spreading branches of trifoliate leaves. The highest quality balsam oil drips from the seeds, but according to biblical scholar Zohar Amar, the balsam extract prepared for the Temple incense was produced by boiling the branches, which have the fragrance of its sap.[17] For production of the incense, the balsam trees had to be cultivated within the boundaries of Israel. It was by far the most expensive and the only tropical spice grown in the Holy Land, always extremely valuable, and literally worth its weight in gold.

According to the first-century AD Jewish historian Josephus, the Queen of Sheba brought the first balsam trees to Israel, as a gift for King Solomon, along with "120 talents of gold, a very great amount of spices, and precious stones."[18] It is also possible that at one time this plant grew wild in the Ein Gedi area, and then was brought under cultivation. The balsam trees were only cultivated and the perfume extracted in three regions of the world, all of them within ancient Israel: at Jericho, at Zoar on the southeastern coast of the Dead Sea, and especially at Ein Gedi on the western shore. Ein Gedi became the most famous area for the production of the rare fragrant oil, identified in the Talmud as being the world famous "Balm of Gilead," referred to in Jeremiah 8:22. Eventually the trees were uprooted by the Romans and became extinct in Israel. According to the Roman historian Pliny, after the destruction of the Temple, the balsam plants were displayed together with the Jewish captives in the triumphal parade through the streets of Rome. It appears that when the Jewish settlement at Ein Gedi was destroyed during stages of the Byzantine Period, the cultivation of balsam there was ended.

The exact processing of the balsam was always a very closely guarded secret. A mosaic tile inscription on the floor of a recently excavated 4th century Ein Gedi synagogue reads: "If anyone reveals the secret of the village to the gentiles, the One whose eyes roam over the entire earth and see what is concealed will uproot this person and his seed from under the sun." The Jews living in this desert oasis wanted to protect their secret recipe for the production of precious balsam perfume. Recent excavations have uncovered one of their ancient workshops for producing balsam oil, including special ovens and vessels. The ancient sages said that the resinous oil has nearly miraculous properties. It heals wounds, is an antidote for snake bites and scorpion stings, and can make a man dizzy with lust. Although the oil was occasionally used as a medicine, more often it was employed as a beautiful incense or perfume. Today this species is nearly extinct worldwide, and until very recently, the only known trees still in existence are cultivated and carefully guarded in the areas of Mecca and possibly Medina, Saudi Arabia.

Balsam is the only fragrance which has its own unique blessing: *boray Shemen Areiv* - Who created the sweet scented oil. The Babylonian amora Rav composed another special blessing for it, "...Who creates the oil of our land." Admiration was expressed in the Talmud for the balsam of Rabbi Judah haNasi's household, and the household of the emperor.[19] In the Messianic era, the Righteous will "bathe in thirteen rivers of Balsam."[20]

The balsam plant has recently been restored to Israel after 1,500 years. In a conference held in Jerusalem on September 1, 2010, it was revealed for the first time that true Judaic balsam (*Commiphora opobalsamum*), known for its unique perfume and extraordinary medicinal properties, has been successfully grown in Israel, after becoming extinct many hundreds of years ago. The re-establishment of this botanical is the result of research conducted by Professor Zohar Amar of the Department of Israel Studies and Archaeology at Bar-Ilan University, in collaboration with Dr. David Iluz. The original plant was cultivated almost exclusively by the Jews, and was considered to be the symbol of the land of Israel. Professor Amar proved in his research that the tradition of identification of the plant and the use of its perfume (in Egypt and the Arabian Peninsula) was preserved until at least the 18th century.

Many attempts have been made to restore the balsam trees to the land of Israel, and several years ago, a few plants were brought to Ein Gedi which were successfully acclimatized. In addition, Amar and Iluz recently brought the plant to Israel from eastern Africa. The researchers who are cultivating these balsam trees have conducted comprehensive scientific pilot studies on the balsam for the past four years. Their studies include work on cultivating and increasing the crop, the chemical and pharmacological properties of liquid resin, various techniques for producing the perfume, and investigating archaeological finds that have been associated with the balsam. Some of the long-term studies are in various stages of publication, while the researchers hope to make further progress when the necessary funding is available.

Tzipporen remains an enigmatic and as yet unidentified spice of the Temple incense. Over thousands of years, this mystery material has been called by many names, including *Shechelet* and *Tofra* (Hebrew), *Onycha* (Greek), *Dofr-al-Afrit* (Arabic), and Devil's Claw. From chemical analyses of samples taken from the 600 kg of Temple incense that was discovered by Vendyl Jones in 1992, each of the 11 Spices was clearly identified, with the exception of this one mysterious item which has caused the most controversy.

The word *tzipporen* in modern Hebrew has a few meanings, most commonly "clove" and "fingernail." The same word also refers to the carnation flower. Currently there are two major theories concerning its true identity. One opinion holds that this incense spice was clove bud (*Eugenia caryophyllata*). The other major theory is that it was an operculum, a highly aromatic part of the shell of a small Mediterranean snail known as a *chilazon* (*Unguis odorata*). Remarkably, the protective organ of this mollusk does indeed have the shape, texture and appearance of a fingernail. It has been recorded that the shell of the creature is aromatic with a "musk-like scent" because it lives on a diet of Spikenard (also a Temple incense spice). The odiferous shells have been gathered at the Red Sea, among other areas, when the heat has dried up the marshes. This snail is closely related to the sea creature that produces the *tehelet* – the blue dye used to prepare the *tzitzit* - fringes - on a four-cornered Jewish garment. Rashi thought *tzipporen* was an aromatic root, shiny like a fingernail. Certain Rabbis of the Talmudic period described onycha as a bitter sap or resin which resembled the shape of a fingernail, from a tree in the myrrh family. Other sages have identified *tzipporen* as rock rose (cistus or labdanum), a shrub with a strong musky scent whose flower petals display fingernail-like markings at their base.

According to the great Kabbalist Alsheikh, looking at our fingernails in the light of the *Havdalah* candle at the end of the Sabbath reenacts Adam looking back at the shining gates of Eden, right after he was expelled from the Garden. The blurred reflection of the light is meant to teach us that no matter how distanced we become from Paradise, we must never forget its luminescence and clarity. Once we have experienced the true light of the Sabbath, any loss of its brilliance can only be temporary.[21] The *tzipporen* is characterized in the Kaballah as being somehow connected with the "clothing" of the first man, before he was expelled from the Garden. Man's original garment of light was said to be smooth like *tzipporen* (fingernails), with the luminescence of pearls, wide below and narrow above.[22] There may be a hint in these teachings regarding "knowledge of the future," which might indicate why the true identity of this spice has so far remained hidden.

Galbanum (*Ferula galbaniflua*) is an extremely foul-smelling tree resin native to Iran. The ten sweet-smelling spices have a lovely fragrance when they are properly combined according to the incense formula. This blend of ten sweet spices, without the galbanum, is over 80% of the mixture, so it would seem that the full blend will still have a fairly nice fragrance even after the galbanum is added. In reality, when the galbanum is finely ground and fully combined into the mixture, something totally miraculous happens: the now complete blend of the eleven spices has *an infinitely more beautiful fragrance* than the ten sweet-smelling spices alone. The galbanum greatly intensifies and more clearly defines the pleasant fragrance of the other ten spices, making the entire incense mixture literally "out of this world." The vileness of the galbanum "flips over" and lifts up the entire blend so it becomes the most beautiful aroma possible, the fragrance of Paradise.

A righteous person is one who grinds the evil within himself so finely that it is completely nullified in the good. The foul-smelling galbanum spice is associated with the evil forces of the world. The eleven spices perfectly combined in the form of the incense therefore represent the complete rectification of evil in this world. The vile galbanum combined within the incense is not only elevated to the level of the other ten blended spices, known as *Kadosh* - Holy; what is much greater, in this process the addition of the galbanum elevates the entire mixture to a much higher level known as *Kodesh Kadoshim* - Holy of Holies.[23] In fact, all of us, except perhaps the most righteous, contain an element of "galbanum" within us, which must be recognized, integrated and uplifted. This great *tikun* – repair - greatly elevates the individual and all of Israel.

Similarly, when those who have wandered away from holiness are brought back into the community, they stand in the very highest spiritual place and in turn raise the entire group to new and previously unimaginable heights. Thus the Talmud says, "Every fast that does not include the sinners of Israel is not (considered in Heaven to be) a (complete and valid) fast!"[24] This is derived from the fact that the incense *must* include the galbanum. Just as the galbanum is necessary, a community on the highest level must include those who have fallen to evil. These fallen sparks must be re-elevated, and returned to the very highest realm of Holiness. The importance of combining all eleven spices is further emphasized by the teaching that an incense maker who left out the galbanum (or any of the other 11 spices) from the mixture would receive the divine death penalty.

Frankincense (*Boswellia carterii*) is also a tree resin that was one of the most prized and costly substances of the ancient world, treasured from the earliest days of civilization, and at times worth its weight in gold. The trees are native to the southern coast of Arabia and Somalia, and also grow abundantly in Ethiopia and India. The fine art of harvesting and processing frankincense has been passed down through the generations. In ancient times, the resin was collected from trees in which cracks had appeared naturally. More recently, to encourage resin production, a deep longitudinal incision is made in the trunk of the tree, and below that a narrow strip of bark about 5" long is peeled off. After two or three weeks, when the milk-like juice which exudes has hardened, the impurities in the wood have been released, and the incision is deepened. In about three months the resin has attained the required consistency, hardening into yellowish drops or "tears." These large globules are then scraped off the tree into baskets. The season for gathering lasts from May until September.

Frankincense has the ability to slow down and deepen the breath, producing feelings of calm which are very conducive to prayer and meditation. It has been burnt on altars and in temples since earliest antiquity. The fragrance is extremely healthy for the entire respiratory system, and treats many ailments such as cough, asthma and chronic bronchitis, as well as skin ailments. It has also been used as a hypnotic perfume in many cosmetics. It is excellent for skin care, particularly in treating the wrinkled skin of the elderly.

Recently it has been shown that the use of frankincense as a medicine may revolutionize the treatment of cancer. Scientists have observed that there is some agent within frankincense which stops cancer from spreading, and which induces cancerous cells to close themselves down. Cancer starts when the DNA code within the cell's nucleus becomes corrupted. Frankincense has a re-set function, and it can tell the cell what the right DNA code should be. It separates the "brain" of the cancerous cell - the nucleus - from the "body" - the cytoplasm, and closes down the nucleus to stop it from reproducing corrupted DNA codes. Currently, with chemotherapy, doctors blast the area around a tumor to kill the cancer, but that also kills healthy cells, and weakens the patient. Treatment with frankincense could eradicate the cancerous cells alone and let the others live.[25]

Levonah zakah - pure frankincense - the most exalted of the *Ketoret* spices, represents the final stage in evolution. A massive awakening will bring the whole world out of a limited awareness that hides the Godly Light, into a totally luminescent state of Messianic consciousness. The frankincense in the incense represents the full revelation of light in the creation, recognizing in everything the *nekuda tovah* - point of holiness – the level of pure white light. Pure frankincense corresponds to the light that surrounds all of the rest of creation.[16] Perhaps this helps to explain why we were commanded to place frankincense around the twelve loaves of holy bread in the Temple: "You shall take the finest grade of wheat flour and bake it into twelve loaves... Arrange (these loaves)... on the undefiled table that is before God (in the Holies). Place pure frankincense alongside these stacks."[26]

Materials used in the preparation of the Incense:

a. "***Borit Karshina***" is lye: 9 *kab* (about 9 quarts – Kaplan). Used for rubbing on the *Tziporren* Spice to refine its appearance.

b. "***Yeyn Kafrisin***" is Cyprus wine: 3 se'in and 3 kab (21 quarts total). Used to steep the *Tziporren* to make its odor more pungent.

c. "***Melach Sedomit***" is Sodom salt: ¼ *kab* (1 cup). Use could contribute to the smoke raising property; certain varieties of salt from this region are rich in potassium, a pyrotechnic ingredient.

d. "***Maaleh Ashan***" is smoke raiser: possibly the herb *Leptadenia pyrotechnica*; another theory is that the three varieties of cinnamon when combined had this effect; or possibly the *Melach Sedomit* **was** the *Maaleh Ashan*. The true identity of this ingredient is still shrouded in mystery.

e. "***Kipat haYarden***" or "Jordan amber" is rose flowers. Rabbi Natan says that a minute quantity was added.

According to Rashi, rose is the true identity of "*Kipat haYarden*," a secret ingredient that was added to the incense mixture. At the end of the Talmud's list of incense ingredients,[27] an extra element called "*Kipat HaYarden*" is mentioned. Rashi says this term literally means "banks of the Jordan," and is a reference to roses that grew along the banks of the Jordan River. There was a time in Jerusalem during the days of the Temple when, except for roses, cultivation of plants was forbidden. No gardens could be planted because of the smells of rot and decay associated with decomposing vegetation and manure that well-tended gardens often produce.[28] Unpleasant odors could not be allowed in the area of God's Sanctuary. Roses on the other hand have the very highest spiritual vibration frequency of any plant or flower, and are thus an excellent choice for uplifting, healing and purification.[29]

Growing roses was permitted in Jerusalem for two reasons, despite the ban. The first reason was tradition: according to the Talmud, there have always been rose gardens in Jerusalem "from the days of the first Prophets." According to Rashi, the other reason that rose gardens - *Ginot Vradim* - were permitted in Jerusalem during Temple times was to cultivate the Jordan River roses that were added to the Temple incense to enhance its fragrance. There is a close correlation between the Hebrew letters in the word *Vradim* – roses - and *Yarden* - Jordan.

Production of the Temple Incense

The yearly cycle of the Ketoret offering began on the first day of *Nisan* and lasted until the end of *Adar*, as this is when the first official offering by Aaron took place. From that day onwards, only a newly produced batch of incense could be used, as it was forbidden to use old Ketoret from the past year until it was mixed into the new batch. Everything that remained behind from the previous year's incense was known as *Motar haKetoret* - leftovers of the incense: 368 *manot* - measures - were produced, but a Jewish Year of 12 months had only 354 days. Thus from a 12 month year there would be 11 measures left over, plus the excess of about 2.5 measures from Yom Kippur - when three manot were brought into the Holy of Holies, although only a large handful was used.

During the production of the new mixture, incense that would be needed to complete the current yearly cycle (right before the first day of the month of Nisan) would be put aside for more immediate use, while the remaining incense would be mixed in with the new batch of 368 measures. Thus the new incense batch would contain a certain amount from previous years (sometimes close to 50% of the total), including some incense that was especially finely ground for past Yom Kippur offerings.

A 12-month lunar year has only 354 days, while a solar year has 365.25 days. The Hebrew calendar combines the lunar and solar cycles. The standard 12-month year follows the lunar cycle, but 7 times in 19 years an extra month of Adar is added – sometimes 29 days, sometimes 30 days – to compensate for the longer 365.25 day sun cycle. With this additional month, the Hebrew calendar and the solar calendars realign perfectly once every 19 years. The Hebrew calendar was given to us by the Holy One at Mt. Sinai through Moses 3,400 years ago, and we have followed it with total accuracy to this day. The Midrash dates it even farther back to the very first days of Adam.[30]

Thus, after every 19-year period, the actual increase of the leftovers was equal to the amount remaining from the past 19 Yom Kippur offerings: about 19 x 2.5 measures or about 47.5 *manot*. Once the leftovers became equal or greater than half the supply needed for the coming year, only a half-batch (184 measures) of new incense would be made. The calculation of when to make only a half-batch of incense had to take into consideration whether the coming year was a 12-month or 13-month year, to insure that there would be enough incense available to reach the first day of Nisan of the coming year.[17]

The incense was prepared by the extremely skillful work of the **Avtinas** (Greek: "a good resin") family of priests, who closely guarded its secrets. They were a clan of highly regarded spice experts who were specially appointed by the Supreme Court for this task, and this family was exclusively responsible for its production. Their secretive craft was performed in their workshop, known as the Chamber of Avtinas, located on the south side of the Temple Courtyard, over the Water Gate. The value of the leftover incense each year was actually the entire salary payment to the Avtinas family for making the incense.

The ownership of the leftover incense was first transferred to the Avtinas family, and then returned by them as a donation to the Temple, in the following way:

1. The left-over Ketoret was theoretically "paid" to the Avtinas family. It's monetary value was then calculated.
2. The equivalent value in money that was due to them was said to increase in holiness, since it was replaced by incense, which temporarily declined in holiness.
3. Money was taken that had been donated as general contributions to the Temple, and it was used to redeem the incense from the Avtinas family, paying their salary. Thus their salary always changed every year, increasing steadily to a great amount over a span of 60 to 70 years, and then diminished to almost zero when a half-batch was made. Then it slowly built up again in value over the next 60 to 70 years.
4. The Avtinas family would then return the leftover incense to the ownership of the Temple, to be mixed together with the newly made batch of incense for the coming year.

The Avtinas family zealously protected the identity of the spices and the exact amounts and manner in which they were prepared. They were particularly secretive about the *Maaleh Ashan* – smoke-rising herb, or more literally "that which causes smoke to rise." It is not clear if the *Maaleh Ashan* was an added ingredient, a special process for preparing the materials, or both. This ingredient and/or process caused the smoke of the incense to rise up to heaven in a straight column. Apparently the Avtinas clan died with this secret, but perhaps it is still hidden away in a sacred writing, waiting to be discovered, or concealed in the "*Pitum HaKetoret*" mystical Incense verses.

Certain passages of the Talmud[31] are very critical of the Avtinas family, focusing on their stubborn refusal to share the knowledge of their craft with others. The same passages also criticize the Bet Garmu family of priests, who were responsible for baking the *Lehem haPanim* - holy bread,32 for keeping their bread-making activities strictly private. In particular, this family would not reveal their secret art of producing beautiful loaves that would not age or mold.

"You (the appointed priests) shall take the finest grade of wheat flour and bake it into twelve loaves... Arrange (these loaves) in two stacks, six loaves to each stack. This shall be placed on the undefiled table that is before God (in the Holies, near the Menorah and incense Altar). Place pure frankincense alongside these stacks. This will be the memorial portion, a fire offering to the Holy One. Every Sabbath day (these loaves) shall be consistently arranged before God. It is an eternal covenant that this must come from the Children of Israel. (This bread) shall be given to Aaron and his descendants, but since it is of the Holy of Holies of God's fire offerings, they must eat it in a sanctified place. This is an eternal law."[33]

In other sources, the secretive nature of the Avtinas and Bet Garmu families is praised.[34] One passage offers an explanation of their behavior: "Our fathers communicated to us their vision that the Temple would eventually be destroyed; should we instruct others in our art, it might come to pass that this knowledge would fall into the wrong hands, and be used in the service of idolatry." Thus such knowledge was always kept as a closely guarded family secret. When the Rabbis understood the reason for their silence, the Avtinas and Bet Garmu families were greatly praised, and are mentioned with reverence as models of scrupulous honesty. It is also taught that no member of the Avtinas family would ever put on perfume. Even when marrying outside of the family, a special agreement was made that the girl would never wear fragrant oils, so that no one would suspect that any member of the family would employ their secret knowledge of the holy incense for personal use.

The Gemara relates[35] that at the height of the criticism of their secretive behavior, both families were removed from their positions. Both families were accused of being too secretive about their work, and requiring too much payment for their services. Expert perfumers and master bakers from Egypt were hired to replace them, and to teach others the long-concealed craft of preparing these holy items. There was concern that key members of the Avtinas and Bet Garmu families might die, and their secret methods might perish with them. Most important, it was expected that the new arrangement would save a significant amount of money, and enrich the Temple treasury, as the Egyptians were content with much smaller salaries. In each case it soon became clear that the Egyptian experts could not match the priestly families. They did not manage to bake holy bread that would not age or become moldy; nor did they succeed in creating a holy incense whose smoke would rise upwards in a straight line to heaven.

Discovering this, the sages and Temple administrators became extremely concerned, because the Ketoret and Show Bread were crucial for the Temple services. They remarked that everything which the Holy One created, He created only for the sake of His own honor. When officials approached the two families to insist upon their immediate return to their positions, the families first conferred, and then agreed that they would resume their responsibilities, based on two conditions: that they would never face the threat of removal again - and that their salaries would be doubled!

Rabbi Akiva related a story told to him by Rabbi Yishmael ben Loga.[36] He was once picking herbs with a descendant of the Avtinas family, who suddenly began to cry, and then laugh. He explained that he had seen the plant that was used to make the Temple incense smoke rise directly upwards. This reminded him of the loss of his family's prestige after the destruction of the Temple, but encouraged him to believe that it would indeed be returned one day in the future. When asked to point out the plant, he refused, saying that his family had sworn never to reveal the secret to others. This story is connected with the theory that the true identity of the *Maaleh Ashan* is the herb *Leptadenia pyrotechnica*, a plant that grows in the southern part of the Jordan Valley and in the northern Sinai. This plant contains nitric acid, ignites very easily, and it has been used to make gunpowder and explosives. A lit branch will burn very quickly, with flames ten meters (over thirty feet) high.

Those who prepared the incense had to know the exact materials to use, and how to purify and process each ingredient before the crucial grinding process was done. Some of the eleven spices needed special advance preparation. The grinding also took great skill, as each spice had to be ground to the same degree of fineness. According to the Rambam, each spice was processed individually. First, each spice would be graded into different sized pieces. For the larger pieces, two huge grinding stones were used to make smaller chunks. The smaller pieces were processed by a *Machtesh*, a special mortar and pestle that had been designed and constructed of brass by Betzalel during the Exodus. It was considered one of the Holy vessels of the Temple, and was ultimately stolen when the Second Temple was plundered. It was known to produce finely ground incense of the very highest quality, and will be difficult to replicate.

The finely ground spice was then slowly put through a series of increasingly fine sifting screens, to achieve a consistent uniform powder. (This process was somewhat similar to the sifting of the fine flour for the *Omer* – barley offering - which was put through a series of 13 progressively finer screens.) What didn't pass through the screens was put back into the *Machtesh*, until the entire material was fully processed. Finally, all of the powdered spices would be mixed together extremely well with Sodom salt, Jordan River rose, and perhaps a smoke-raising herb, to produce the finished incense.

During the actual grinding process, one priest would rhythmically chant, "*Hadak heytev, heytev hadak* - grind it fine, finely grind it," while another priest (or sometimes two or three together) were pulverizing the spices. They would grind in rhythm to the beat of the meditative chant, which invigorated the workers, kept them in high spirits, and kept the grind consistent. Pulverizing the spices raised a lot of dust, and the guttural chant blew air and spice dust safely out of the throat.

Also, the *Machtesh* had bells all around it. Rashi said that the sound of the voices chanting and the bells clinking enriched the incense. Sound waves and vibration are damaging to wine, but beneficial for holy spice processing. This is cross-sensory stimulation, which takes place in altered states of consciousness. Again it must be emphasized that the unique grinding process of the incense is said to have given it special powers to rule over Death and elevate a person to the exalted level of Prophecy.

Offering the Incense

The Temple incense was to be burned only on the *Mizbayach Zahav* - golden incense altar, made of acacia wood overlaid with beaten gold. A valuable timber tree, acacia is very hard and close-grained, uniting the qualities of strength and durability. According to the Midrash, Jacob brought acacia trees with him to Egypt, and had them planted in Goshen. He did this so that when the Israelites would leave Egypt hundreds of years later, they would cut these trees down and bring them along for use in building the Tabernacle.[37] The exact construction and use of this altar was taught to Moses on Mt. Sinai, and this revelation appears in the written Torah:

"Make an altar of acacia wood to burn incense. It shall be rectangular, a cubit (an "*Ama*" – the distance from the elbow to the fingertips) long and a cubit wide, and two cubits high, including its horns" (18" x 18" x 36," and some say 15" x 15" x 30"). Some think it was solid wood, and some say it was an inverted box. Some say the "horns" were small cubes 2.25" on each corner, and others say they were horn-like protrusions. "Cover it with a layer (as thick as a dinar) of pure gold, on its top, its walls all around, and its horns. Make a gold rim all around it. Place two gold rings under (the altar's) rim on its two opposite sides as receptacles to hold the poles with which it is carried." Some say the two rings were on opposite corners; others say it had four rings, one on each corner. "Make the carrying poles of acacia wood and cover them with a layer of gold. Place (this altar) in front of the cloth partition (between the table and the lamp) concealing the Testimony Ark – before the cloth partition, concealing the Testimony area where I commune with you. Aaron shall burn incense on (this altar) each morning when he cleans out the lamps. He shall (also) burn (incense) before evening when he lights the lamps. Thus, for all generations, there will be incense before God at all times. Do not burn any unauthorized incense" (donated by an individual, or made with unauthorized ingredients) "on it. Furthermore, do not offer any animal sacrifice, meal offering or libation on it. (Furthermore), once each year Aaron shall make atonement (by placing blood) on the horns of (this altar). For all generations, he shall make atonement with the blood of the atonement sacrifice once each year (on Yom Kippur). (This altar) shall be a Holy of Holies to God."[38]

Even the task of bringing the coals for the incense offering, done by another priest chosen by the lottery, was a coveted assignment. The lottery system was established, as many Cohanim wanted the honor of offering Ketoret or bringing the coals. It is said that Cohanim would even fight over the opportunity to empty and clean out the *ashes of the coals* after the incense was consumed! We learn that this was a revered task, and many priests used every persuasive device to receive this special honor.

On the outer altar there were three separate fire pits: One for the main altar, for the animal sacrifices; one to produce coals for the daily offerings of the Ketoret; and one to produce coals for the Yom Kippur offering, to be used only once each year. It was very important that the coals for the Ketoret offerings would burn cleanly, without producing smoke, sparks or sounds. Trees for these fires would need to be cut before Tu B'Av, so they would dry properly. Twelve different types of trees were used for the fires, and most contained aromatic oils. Fig was considered the best wood to use, while olive and grapevine wood were never used, due to excessive smoke, moisture or knots. No wounded, old, or wormy wood was permitted.

Weather conditions did not affect the fires on the altar. Miraculously, rain or wind would not cause any changes in the burning or coal production. It is also considered a miracle that the incense altar stayed in perfect condition and lasted so long, since there were two fires on it every day. Clumps of the burning incense which fell from the coals on the altar onto the sides or floor could not be retrieved or touched. These would be cleaned up later by the priests who had the privilege of emptying the ashes from the incense altar.

On Yom Kippur, the High Priest [*Color Plates 14 & 15 – the High Priest*] would offer the Temple incense three times: twice upon the golden incense altar in the Sanctuary, as was done every day, and once in the Holy of Holies. Taking a gold fire pan, the High Priest climbed the outer (animal sacrifice) altar, and filled the pan with coals from a specially designated fire on the altar's southwest corner. Next, the High Priest was brought a small shovel full containing 3 Measures of incense from the Avtinas Chamber, pouring it into a special golden vessel. (According to Rabbi Aryeh Kaplan, one Measure is about 5 lbs.) He then took the golden vessel in his left hand and the pan of coals in his right, and made his way to the Sanctuary.

When the High Priest reached the Ark of the Covenant, he set down the pan with the burning coals between the two poles at the base of the Ark. Now the High Priest was called upon to perform the most difficult task in his entire service: pouring the incense from the golden vessel into his own hands. To do this he would clasp the vessel with his fingertips or teeth, and using his thumbs, would pour the incense into his palms taking a double handful of fragrant mixture, without spilling a drop. He would then pile the incense on top of the coals in the fire pan, creating a thick column of smoke.

In the days of the Second Temple, the original Ark of the Covenant was missing from the Holy of Holies. Just before the First Temple was destroyed, Jeremiah hid it until the end of days. According to the Mishna, a stone called the *Evven Shetiyah* – Foundation Stone, the Eye of the Universe, had been there since the days of the early Prophets. This stone was three fingerbreadths high, and the gold fire pan was placed here. The Holy of Holies was built upon the *Evven Shetiyah*, and the world was established on this precise Center-Point of Planet Earth.[39] This was the very first point at which God began the creation of the physical universe,[40] and from this point the universe unfolded until the Holy One decreed that it should stop.[41] The *Sefer Yetzira* places the Foundation Stone at a central place in Hebrew cosmology as the stone that God flung into the abyss to form matter and creation. Some traditions hold that the *Evven Shetiyah* actually served as the altar in the Temple, and that at its base were the pits that God drilled from the surface of the earth to the depths below, connecting the "waters above to the waters below."

Rabbi Aryeh Kaplan brings many sources which provide valuable information concerning the Foundation Stone, showing that it is the interface between the Spiritual dimension and the physical world.[42] This is the exact mid-point between the two *Kruvim* - Cherubim or Angels - that stood on top of the Ark of the Covenant, the focal point of all prophetic inspiration, even though the Ark and Cherubim miraculously did not take up any physical space.[43] "When Moses entered the *Ohel Moed* – Communion Tent – to speak with Him, he would hear the Voice speaking to him *from between the two Angels* that are upon the Ark of Testimony."[44]

On Yom Kippur, when the Ketoret was offered in the *Kodesh Kadoshim*, the burning would create a "smoke screen" between the *Cohen Gadol* - High Priest - and the *Aron Kodesh* - Holy Ark. The High Priest must not see the Shechina hovering over the Angels above the Ark Cover, so he would not die. A verse in the Torah says: "There, before God, he shall place the incense on the fire, so that the smoke from the incense hides his view of the Ark cover, over the (Tablets of) Testimony. Then he will not die."[45] This is the primary reason for the inclusion of the *Maaleh Ashan* - smoke-raising herb, to create a separation for the Cohen Gadol's protection.

The *Tz'dukim* – Sadducees - debated with the *Hachamim* - wise men – about where exactly to light the incense on Yom Kippur. The Sadducees held that it should be put onto the coals *outside* of the Holy of Holies by the High Priest, and then brought inside already smoking. The wise men who were the authorities in charge absolutely insisted that he should enter with the fire pan (coals) in his right hand, the Ketoret in a golden vessel in his left hand, and put the Ketoret onto the coals *only once he is inside* the Holy of Holies, right at the base of the Holy Ark of the Covenant. The authorities would make certain that a Sadducee High Priest would take an oath to do things *their* way. The wise men saw the Ketoret sacrifice as the most important ceremony and the main part of the Holy work on Yom Kippur, and this is why they felt that it should be burned only *inside* the Holy of Holies. Perhaps the Sadducees were correct. Igniting the incense before entering the Holy of Holies would provide an important smoke screen that was required to completely block any view of the Ark.

Forbidden Things

Only a true Cohen who is a direct descendant of Aaron is permitted to offer the incense. Anyone who is not from this family, including even the King of Israel, is considered an *ish zar* - strange man, meaning a non-priest, and is strictly forbidden to offer Ketoret at any time or engage in other priestly functions. The actual sin of Aaron's sons Nadav and Avihu may have been that they burned Ketoret in the Holy of Holies like the High Priest on Yom Kippur, and even though they were both priests, for this unauthorized use they left this world. There are other widely varying opinions about this. It was known that the Ketoret smoke of a true Cohen, whose Offering is accepted by the Holy One, would always rise straight upwards, although this did not minimize the importance of properly including the "smoke riser" in the incense.

If an incense maker (or anyone else) placed honey in the incense, it was unfit for sacred use. Rabbi Bar Kappara taught that if a minute quantity of honey had been mixed into the Ketoret, a man could not stand up straight because of the fragrance, and no one could have resisted the scent. The Torah states: "No leaven or honey shall be burned as a fire offering to God. Do not make any meal offering that is sacrificed to God out of leavened dough. This is because you may not burn anything fermented or sweet as a fire offering. Although these may be brought as a first-fruit offering (which was not placed on the altar), they may not be offered on the altar as an appeasing fragrance."[46] *Devash* in Hebrew is usually translated as "honey." Here, it denotes any type of fruit juice,[47] especially date extract.[48] Others take this more literally to mean bee's honey.

Honey and leaven both allude to pride, which is hateful to God. These materials rise as if they have pride in themselves. The Torah teaches that whatever "bubbles and expands" when heated represents *ta'avah* – lust - and *ga'avah* - vanity). This is why anything fermented or sweet is forbidden as a fire offering.[16]

It is forbidden to formulate the incense for personal use, or make any use of the incense for personal enjoyment. At its core, the Temple incense is dedicated entirely to the Holy One, to fulfill His Commandment, even though we people greatly benefit from it. Those who violate this prohibition have the Judgment of *Karet* (being spiritually cut off from one's ancestors). This is a great loss especially if one's ancestors are people who were highly esteemed by God. For educational purposes or to help the congregation, one is exempt from the death penalty, but if he violates the prohibition under these circumstances, during the days of the Temple he would be required to bring a *Korban M'ilah* – misappropriation offering - to atone for this more minor transgression. Even the incense makers, the Avtinas family, would carefully observe this prohibition: during production of the incense they would plug up their noses, so they wouldn't inadvertently smell and enjoy the fragrances. This prohibition includes producing the actual incense, but it does *not apply* to using or blending the essential oil extracts of the eleven incense spices, since no grinding is involved in producing or blending them.

It is forbidden to enjoy the first moment of the Ketoret burning, even for the priest doing the offering or other priests inside the Temple. This shows respect and the awareness that the incense is dedicated entirely to the Holy One. When the Priest first lit the Ketoret he would shout out, and the other Priests in the area would hold their noses, so they would not violate this prohibition. In addition, Saadia Gaon taught that there are three specific places inside the Temple where it is forbidden to smell the incense burning: In the *Heichal* – inner chamber of the Temple, in the Ulam – domed foyer, and in the area between the *Ulam* and the *Mizbayach* – incense altar. Whenever the incense was lit, the other priests would clear out of these Holy places inside the Temple. After the actual burning they were permitted to return, even though these areas were still filled with beautiful fragrance.

Mystical Incense Recitation

Over the past two thousand years since the final days of the Second Temple, the recitation of the mystical verses regarding the Temple incense offering known as "*Pitum HaKetoret*" has temporarily replaced the actual offering, until the time when the Temple will be restored. As we have learned, more than the other sacrifices, the incense offering *is always* standing before the Holy One throughout all generations. In other words, it is not just limited to the days of the Temple; this special connection to God is always accessible to all of us. Elijah the Prophet came to teach Rabbi Pinchas that during these days of exile when there is no Temple, reciting these verses with true intention and deep concentration has the very same healing power as the priest offering incense in the Temple on the golden altar. One must learn and understand the true meaning of the words, and then he can know exactly what he is saying (and doing) when he reads these verses. He is regarded in Heaven just as if he is actually performing the Temple incense sacrifice exactly in the way that it is meant to be done.

The word "*Pitum*" has the connotation of "mixing up" or "blending," of being an alchemist. Through the proper recitation of these verses, we are credited as if we personally offered the incense,[49] and as a result we are protected from all harm. The Temple incense, and even the recitation, breaks the power of the evil inclination from all sides. According to the Zohar, smelling the incense as it rose from the altar would purify the heart of the priest making the offering, instilling clarity and love, and imbuing him with the will to serve his Master. Consciously reciting these verses has the same effect. The impurity left by the evil inclination will be lifted from him, and he will have One Heart devoted to the Holy One.[50]

Anyone who reads these verses every day with true intention and clarity is saved from magic spells, evil occurrences, evil thinking, evil judgment and death. Whoever says them slowly each day without skipping a word, and understands what he is saying, is protected against all evil occurrences and evil thoughts, and from an evil death. He can rest assured that he will not be harmed in any way; he will be protected from punishments, and will have a portion in the World to Come. When *Pitum HaKetoret* has not been recited with devotion, judgments from above can dwell upon him, there can be a great plague, and other nations can rule over him. Rabbi Shimon Bar Yochai said: "If people knew how great it is when they recite the section of *Pitum HaKetoret* before the Holy One, they would take every word and place it on their heads like a golden crown!"

Saying these verses with total consciousness will help a person repair himself in every way, and return to complete purity and holiness. It is written, "He will count the eleven *Simanim* (referring to both the incense spices, and the *Sefirot*) on his fingers, know the meaning of each one, and through this will be able to say the verses with full concentration. Doing so, according to the depth of focus and one's merit, increases the power of the words, allowing them to elevate these eleven Aspects of Holiness to their Source."[51] Rabbi Moshe Ben Yehuda Machir z"l, who was among the great Rabbis of Tzfat during the time of Rabbi Yitzhak Luria, said: "One who has concern for himself and his soul should expend all of his efforts regarding this matter…read it in the morning and evening with great concentration, and I will be his guarantor."[52]

Elijah the Prophet is said to assist in this and every heavenly transmission, and he is one of the "eight princes among men"[53] whose lifetimes span all of world history.[54] When the heavenly court finds the world worthy of being shaken, Elijah stands and reminds the court of the merit of the Patriarchs, and then God has mercy on His world.[55] It is written that he was privileged to be able to revive the dead, because he did the will of the Holy One, Blessed be He.[56] According to the Rambam, Elijah the Prophet will need to re-appear before the arrival of the Messiah,[57] and this means that prophecy will be reinstated in the world.[58]

Elijah taught Rabbi Pinchas what to do in the event of a plague. The Holy One made a covenant in Heaven with the destroying Angel, that if a community gathers together to say the *Pitum HaKetoret* with true intention, the plague will be nullified. This is a story from the Zohar about Rabbi Acha, and how he stopped a plague through the recitation of *Pitum HaKetoret*:

Rabbi Acha went to visit the village of Tarsha, where there had been a severe plague for seven days, and it was getting worse every day. This is an indication of immoral and corrupt behavior. His intention was to help people to mend their ways and return to God. At first he suggested that everyone come to the House of Worship to pray, but then he realized that this was not a time for prayer - the situation was too severe. He instructed the villagers to gather forty of the most righteous people available. They would divide into four groups, one at each corner of the village, and chant the verses of *Pitum HaKetoret* with deep concentration three times, asking the Holy One for mercy. After this, the righteous people went to the homes of people who were ill, and said *Pitum HaKetoret* there, followed by the verses from the Torah in which Aaron is instructed by Moses to carry the burning Temple incense through the camp to stop the plague of death:

"Moses then said to Aaron, 'Take the fire pan and place on it some fire from the altar. Offer incense and go quickly to the community to make atonement for them. Divine wrath is coming forth from God. The plague has already begun!' Aaron took (the pan) as Moses had told him, and ran to the middle of the assembled masses, where the plague had already begun to kill the people. He offered the incense to atone for them. As he stood between the dead and the living, the plague was checked."[59]

Then Rabbi Acha and the community heard a heavenly Voice saying, "the Secret of Secrets is being revealed here, the secret that the Angel of Death revealed to Moses!" Then the villagers said, "Even the judgment of Heaven can not dwell here, because now we know how to nullify it." Afterwards, Rabbi Acha became weak. He felt that not everyone had mended their ways. He dozed off, and it was revealed to him that his strength and power had indeed ended the plague, and he was able to facilitate this because the manifestation of evil did not affect him. Now his task was to help all the people of this village overcome evil and mend their ways. He did so. The people of that village did a complete fixing, and made a commitment to study Torah and observe the ways of the Holy One. They then changed the name of that village from Tarsha to *Mata Machatzia* - the Holy One had mercy on us.

There are many great benefits to reading the verses of *Pitum HaKetoret*, especially when they are read with kavanna - deep concentration - from a kosher parchment, written with Ashurite lettering – the same letter forms that are used to write a *Sefer Torah, Megillas Ester, Tefillin* or *Mezuzah*. According to Rabbi Pinchas Zevichi, "it follows that one who reads the *Pitum HaKetoret* from a kosher parchment will certainly be blessed from heaven with healthy children, a comfortable livelihood, with riches and happiness, and will be successful in all areas, as well as in his spiritual growth. Thus, it will be beneficial for him and his children forever. It will be a *segula* - good sign - for the protection and salvation of all of Israel, and the merit of the *klal* – community - will be derived from him."[60]

Although Rabbi Zevichi's statement specifically mentions men, we have found no indication from our sources that a proper reading by any of our holy women would be any less effective for them. During Temple days, this very special "incense connection" was made only by a specially chosen priest. Today it appears to be equally available to *everyone*.

The following is stated in the Sefer "*Kaf HaChaim*" written by the Gaon Rabbi Chaim Pelagie: "One should write the Ketoret on a parchment in Ashurite lettering as in a Torah scroll, and read from this parchment; it is a great *segula* – good omen - as the Ketoret brings wealth. He is promised that his livelihood will be plentiful and he will be able to live a very comfortable life."[61] In his book *Ruach Chaim* on the *Shulchan Aruch* he adds "reading the Ketoret from Ashurite lettering on a parchment as in a Sefer Torah is a *segula* for wealth, and will bring him success in all of his business affairs."[62]

Most *Ashkenazim* – Jews of northwestern Europe - say the *Pitum HaKetoret* twice per day, at the beginning and end of the Morning Service. Among the *Sefardim* – Jews of southern Europe, North Africa and Asia - the custom is to say *Pitum HaKetoret* three times every day. These present-day readings are intended to parallel and temporarily replace the actual Temple practices, in their original order. The first recitation is at the beginning of the morning service, right after saying the portion dealing with the daily sacrifice (known as "*Tamid*"). This is in place of the incense that was burned in the Temple every morning. Next, the *Pitum HaKetoret* is said by the Sefardim at the end of the morning prayers. This is a remedy against the destructive nature of the "Other Side," and has the power to annul any evil forces that would denounce the prayers. This recitation can even remedy the entire Service. Finally, it is said again before the afternoon service - *Mincha*, corresponding to the late afternoon incense burning. Many people have the custom of saying the *Pitum HaKetoret* on Saturday night after *Havdallah*, the ceremony that concludes the Sabbath. This reading has great power to nullify evil, and it brings success to a person in everything he does throughout the week.

Translation of the Mystical Incense Recitation by Rabbi Avraham Sutton:

"You are the Lord our God and God of our fathers before whom our ancestors burned the offering of incense when the Temple stood, as You have commanded them through Moses Your Prophet, as it is written in your Torah:

'The Lord said to Moses: Take fragrant spices, balsam, *tziporren* (possibly clove or snail shell), and galbanum, fragrant spices, and pure frankincense; there shall be an equal weight of each. And you shall make it into incense, a compound expertly blended, well-mingled, pure and holy. You shall grind some of it very fine, and put some of it (only on Yom Kippur) before the Ark in the Tabernacle, where I will meet with you; most Holy shall it be to you.[63] And it is written: Aaron shall burn upon the altar the incense of fragrant spices; every morning when he cleans the lamps (of the Menorah), he shall burn it. And toward evening, when Aaron lights the Menorah, he shall burn it; this is a *continual* incense offering before the Lord *throughout your generations*.'[64]

The Rabbis have taught:[65] How was the incense prepared? It weighed 368 measures: 365 corresponding to the number of days in the solar year, one measure for each day – half a measure to be offered in the morning and half toward evening; and the other three measures (are those) from which the High Priest took two handfuls (into the Holy of Holies) on Yom Kippur. These (three measures) were put back into the mortar on the day before Yom Kippur and ground again very thoroughly so as to make the incense extremely fine. The incense contained the following eleven kinds of spices: balsam, *tziporen*, galbanum, frankincense – each one weighing seventy measures; myrrh, cassia, spikenard, saffron – each weighing sixteen measures; Costus, twelve measures; Aromatic Bark, three (measures); Cinnamon, nine (measures). (Also used in the preparation of the incense were): lye of Carshina, nine *kabin*; Cyprus wine, three se'in and three kabin – if Cyprus wine was not available, strong white wine might be used instead; salt of Sodom, a fourth of a *kab*; and a minute quantity of a smoke-raising herb. Rabbi Nathan the Babylonian says: A minute quantity of *Kipat HaYarden* - Jordan amber, quite possibly rose flowers - was also added. If, however, honey was added, the incense became unfit; while if one left out any of the ingredients, he was liable to the death penalty.

Rabbi Shimon ben Gamliel says: The balsam is none other than the resin which exudes from the (Judaic) balsam trees. The lye of Carshina was used for rubbing on the Tziporen to refine its appearance. The Cyprus wine was used to steep the Tziporen to make its odor more pungent. Though the water of *Raglayim* (urine?) might have served that purpose well, it would be disrespectful to bring it into the Temple.

It has been taught, Rabbi Nathan says: "While the priest was grinding the incense, the overseer would chant, 'grind it fine, grind it fine,' because the (rhythmic) sound (of the voice) is good for the compounding of the spices." If only half the required yearly quantity of incense was prepared, it was fit for use; but we have not heard if it was permissible to prepare only a third or a fourth of it. Rabbi Yehudah said: "The general rule is that if the incense was compounded in its correct proportions, it was fit for use even if only half the annually required quantity was prepared; if, however, one left out any of its ingredients, he was liable to the death penalty."

It has been taught, Bar Kappara says: "Once in sixty or seventy years, half of the required yearly quantity of incense came from the accumulated surpluses (from the three measures from which the High Priest took two handfuls on Yom Kippur every year)." Bar Kappara also taught: Had a minute quantity of honey been mixed into the incense, no one could have resisted the scent. Why then was no honey mixed with it? This is because the Torah says: "You shall present neither leaven nor honey as an offering by fire to the Lord."[66]

These verses from Psalms are recited at the end of the reading:

Salvation is the Lord's; Your Blessing is upon Your people, Selah.[67]

The Lord of hosts is with us; the God of Jacob is our stronghold forever.[68] (Said three times)

Lord of hosts, happy is the man who trusts in you.[69] (Said three times)

Lord, deliver us; may the King answer us on the day we call.[70] (Said three times)

May the Offering of Judah and Jerusalem be pleasing to the Holy One as in the days of old, and as in former years.[71]

Personal incense offerings

***Tikkun Chatzot* – The Midnight Repair.** The recitation of *Pitum HaKetoret* can be an important element within the mystic ritual of the *Tikkun Chatzot*, a special devotional service that is begun precisely in the middle of the night. Although this practice is well known as a pathway to mourning the destruction of the Temple, its ancient roots are far more obscure. It is said that at this time, the Holy Blessed One enters the Garden of Eden to rejoice with His Creation. The ritual, meditation and visualizations of *Tikkun Chatzot* are designed to bring us to a state of consciousness in which we can tap into this divine energy, and draw it back into our world. It is a bridge from the Garden of Eden to our earthly plane, of Creation-consciousness infused into the ordinary world, and an attempt to grasp the mind of the Holy One. This encounter with God becomes a thread of grace which we carry with us into our day, and with which we actively bridge and bind night and day together with holiness.

Tikkun Chatzot is a mystic journey in which we experience the death and release of the soul from the body as a way to approach God intimately. As we approach, we grasp God consciousness at the moment of creation, when the Holy One is rejoicing in His Garden. We also enter the Garden and rejoice, and this is followed by a rebirth as the soul is drawn back into the body. As we return, carrying the whisper of this encounter with God consciousness, the spices and incense of the Garden also return with us. "Awake, North Wind, and come you South. Blow in my garden that the incense may float out."[72] The aroma of the Garden and the incense are critical elements. Thus it may be very helpful and beneficial to burn incense during the ceremony. The aroma activates our ability to grasp creation consciousness, and incense is the mystic element which mediates the forces of creation while we go through the ritual of visioning, dying and re-birthing. An important key is to begin this ritual at the exact mid-point of the night, when God is entering and will be present in the Garden of Eden.[73]

We find evidence that in ancient times, various types of permitted personal incense were commonly used, as many stone or porcelain square-based incense burners were found in excavations. The older models had points on the corners, similar to the *Mizbayach Zahav* - golden Temple incense altar. Kings of Israel had specially built incense altars of their own, but they were strictly forbidden to offer the Temple incense on their personal altars, or even in the Temple – a privilege that was reserved exclusively for priests.

Some other occasions for burning personal incense:

1. For enjoyment and health care, and to lift your energy level. Especially mentioned is burning the resins of frankincense and myrrh at night;
2. to bring a good fragrance to a person's place of work;
3. as a prevention against the *Ayin HaRah* – "evil eye";
4. to heal plagues and repel insects;
5. for spiritual ceremonies such as weddings, and on days of mourning;
6. as *Moogmar*, a dessert offering after a meal, especially when entertaining special guests. It can bring an absolutely beautiful fragrance to the home, and is ignited just after the *Bircas HaMazon* - blessings after a meal;
7. on the eve of festivals or the Sabbath;
8. to cleanse clothes and dishes;
9. to preserve respect, and purify the scent of a deceased body before burial;
10. to cleanse and purify the air and environment at any time, and elevate consciousness.

Some authorities teach us to say a blessing on personal incense at the time when it is lit, as long as it is a natural fragrance and causes smoke. Some say it is best to not make a Blessing on various types of incense that are or were used for *avoda zara* - idol worship. This is not to be taken lightly, as it is closely related to the Second Commandment.

Food for Thought

There is a close relationship between the food we eat, our thoughts and actions, and our sacrificial offerings at the Temple. Similar to the galbanum, whenever a harsh punishment has been decreed against us because of some evil deed, this very evil must be elevated. Since the Original Sin occurred when Adam and Eve ate from the "Tree of Knowledge," one major rectification in living a holy life is through fasting. An even greater ultimate fixing is learning to eat properly and with a much higher consciousness.

When we eat and digest food with the primary intention of serving the Creator, the food is converted into positive energy, and our body chemistry actually gives forth a *rayach nichoach* – sweet fragrance. Having been nourished by the sanctified food, our body engaged in good deeds gives off a lovely aroma. Conversely, if the food energy is used to do evil, our chemistry gives forth an unpleasant odor. Thus eating food is analogous to the sacrifices on the Temple altar: The "fire" of our digestive system is compared to the fire on the altar, and our digestive process hopefully elevates the sparks of life in the food. A person's body is like a microcosm of the whole world. Every limb has the potential to fix or complete a flaw or lack in the universe. Since we have no Temple today, our prayers have replaced the sacrifices, including the incense offering. In deep prayer, the soul infuses the body with energy, and consciousness becomes totally present and permeates each cell of our being.

Some Rabbinic scholars, including Rabbi Kook *z"l*, contend that in the Third Temple there won't be any animal sacrifices at all, and the primary sacrifice will be the incense offering. This opinion is based on the language of the passage following the *Shemoneh Esrei Amidah* (the silent prayer that is meditated three times each day), in which we say: "*V'ahrvah laShem* ***Minchat*** *Yehudah v'Yerushalayim kimay olam u-ch'shanim kadmoniyot,*" which means "then the Offering of Judah and Jerusalem will be pleasing to God, as in days of old and in former years." The Mincha Service in the Temple was composed of only a meal offering and incense, and since the prayer specifically mentions *Mincha*, Rav Kook deduces that the offerings in the Third Temple will include the incense offering, but not involve any animal sacrifices.[73]

This interpretation by Rabbi Kook implies that at the End of Days we will no longer need the intermediary step of placing an animal between ourselves and God. The great Torah commentator Nachmanides taught that in the Third Temple we will all be vegetarians. This parallels the teaching of Rabbi Kook above. A nation that sacrifices animals on the Temple altar may eat meat, but in the future when we no longer sacrifice animals in the Temple, we will no longer consume them within the human "altar" of our body and digestive system.

Chapter 4

Anointing Oil: the Divine Perfume

In March 1988, Dr. Vendyl Jones and his team of Noahide volunteers found a clay jug measuring approximately five inches high in a cave at Qumran, just northwest of the Dead Sea. Jones is a Biblical Archeologist who had been excavating the area for over 20 years, based on information decoded from the ancient Copper Scroll of Jeremiah, and other rabbinic sources. The jug he discovered in a carefully planned archaeological search contained very unusual oil. It was identified as genuine *Shemen haMishchah* – anointing oil of Moses - that was prescribed in the Torah for anointing the Tabernacle and its vessels, as well as certain priests and kings of Israel. The oil was still viscous, but because it was several thousand years old, it had solidified into a gelatin-like substance that resembles molasses. The vessel that contained the oil was wrapped in palm leaves, and carefully concealed in a 3-foot-deep pit that protected it from looting and preserved it during the extreme climate changes of the area. This jug is currently on display at the Israel Museum, and its contents were tested and then sealed and placed in a refrigerated vault in the pharmaceutical department of Hebrew University.[1]

During the revelation of the Torah on Mt. Sinai, Moses received the commandment to produce one complete batch of anointing oil, dedicated entirely to the Holy One, to last for all Eternity. According to Biblical sages Rashi and Sforno, the anointing oil made by Moses will remain forever, and will never need to be produced again. Concurrently, one of the 613 commandments of the Torah divinely decreed to all of the people of Israel was to insure that the anointing oil would be used exactly as God commanded Moses. The oil is considered extremely holy, and must be employed only according to God's command. According to Maimonides, the Holy One proclaimed that the anointing oil is "for Me," and is only in the custody of the priests, but is not owned by them.

The Torah informs us: "God spoke to Moses, saying: Take the finest spices, 500 (*shekels* weight) of distilled myrrh, (two) half portions, each consisting of 250 (*shekels*) of fragrant cinnamon and 250 (*shekels*) of *Keneh Bosem*, and 500 (*shekels*) of cassia, all measured by the Sanctuary standard, along with a *hin* of olive oil. Make (these materials) into a sacred Anointing Oil. Blend it (all) into a compound, as made by a master perfumer...

"Then use (this blend) to anoint the Communion Tent, the Ark of Testimony, the Table and all its utensils, the Menorah and its utensils, the Incense Altar, the sacrificial altar and all its utensils, the Washstand and its base. You will thus sanctify them, making them Holy of Holies, so that anything touching them becomes sanctified. You must also anoint Aaron and his sons (with this Oil), sanctifying them as priests to Me.

"Speak to the Israelites, and tell them: this shall be the sacred anointing oil to Me for all generations. Do not pour it on the skin of any (unauthorized) person, and do not duplicate it with a similar formula. It is Holy, and it must remain sacred to you. If a person blends a similar formula, or places it on an unauthorized person, he shall be cut off (spiritually) from his people."[2]

The Anointing Oil had three purposes:

1. To consecrate the holy vessels of the Tabernacle in the desert, once and for all time;
2. To anoint the first High Priest, Aaron HaCohen, and every High Priest after him,[3] as well as the Priest of War;[4]
3. To anoint King David and the later Kings of his dynasty, whenever their right to the royal throne is in dispute.[5]

The anointing oil and the Temple incense are deeply connected. Both have four major ingredients specified in the written Torah; both are considered to be *Kodesh Kadoshim* - Holy of Holies; the punishment for producing or misusing the anointing oil or Temple incense, or employing them for private use – especially to personally enjoy the fragrance, is "*Karet*" - being spiritually cut off from the Jewish people.[6]

This is the recipe for the anointing oil as it appears in the written Torah, with the amounts shown in *shekels* weight (500 *shekels* equals about 25 lbs.):

a. 500 ***Mar Dror***: "pure" myrrh (probably distilled myrrh oil)

b. 500 ***Kinman Besem***: fragrant cinnamon bark, in 2 portions of 250 *shekels* each

c. 250 ***Keneh Bosem***: this could be calamus, lemongrass or palmarosa; Rabbi Aryeh Kaplan thinks it was cannabis.[7]

d. 500 ***Kidah***: Cassia (Chinese cinnamon)

e. 1 *hin* (12 "*logs*" or about 3-4 liters) of ***Shemen Zayit***: olive oil (V. Jones: jojoba oil)

We do not know with certainty which ingredients Moses used to make the anointing oil. In particular, there are varying opinions about the true botanical identity of *Keneh Bosem*, and chemical analyses of the ancient oil found by Vendyl Jones were not conclusive. Although the Torah seems to stipulate the use of olive oil as the carrier, according to Dr. Jones the anointing oil was made by cooking the spices into Jojoba oil, not olive oil. In his opinion, Moses knew that only jojoba oil, which is native to Israel, would preserve the anointing oil for all time. As evidence of this, Jones points out that the anointing oil was also known as *Shemen HaTov* - the "good oil." In fact olive oil should not be used as a perfume carrier as it is prone to spoilage and rancidity, whereas jojoba oil has an unlimited shelf life and is a perfect carrier for the best perfumes.

Producing the anointing oil and the Temple incense were the very first tasks Moses was to attend to after he descended from Mt. Sinai. He made the anointing oil as follows: Moses crushed each spice separately, similar to the Ketoret process, and then he blended the spices together and soaked the mixture in pure, sweet-tasting water until their aroma was completely absorbed. He then added the carrier oil, and cooked the blend down over an open flame until all the water was boiled off. After he filtered out the debris, only the pure anointing oil remained. Another opinion, similar to Jones, is that the spices were cooked directly in the carrier oil without using any water, and then all of the remaining debris was filtered out.[8]

Only 4 of the 11 spice ingredients of the Temple incense are mentioned in the written Torah, whereas most authorities believe that the entire recipe appears for the anointing oil. According to our sages, this indicates that when the anointing oil was made, only the *full recipe amount* could be produced, and only one time by Moses. However, for the Temple incense, a full recipe, half-recipe or partial recipe could be produced as many times as needed, as long as the primary ingredients were used in the same relative proportions. Some authorities maintain that although the four spices named in the Torah were the main ingredients of the anointing oil, it also contained small amounts of all eleven spices that were used to make the Temple incense.

A total of 12 *logs* of anointing oil was produced and stored by Moses in 24 half-*log* sealed jugs. The first one was used to anoint all of the Holy Vessels of the Tabernacle, and the High Priest Aaron HaCohen. The second jug was used to anoint his son Elazar when he arose to become the High Priest. The third one was used for over a thousand years to anoint the succeeding High Priests, and also King David and some of his lineage. This is the vessel that was discovered by Vendyl Jones in 1988. The remaining 21 sealed jugs were hidden away inside the Ark of the Covenant seven years before the destruction of the First (Solomon's) Temple, when Priests and Levites responded to Jeremiah's prophecy of impending doom. This highly secretive task was carried out in 593 BCE at the command of King Josiah, because of Jeremiah's revelation that the Temple treasures must be hidden away and recovered only for use in the Third Temple, in the Messianic period known as the "End of Days." For this reason the Temple treasures were not excavated during the 420 years of the Second Temple, even though the hidden location was known to some of the elders.

The Anointment of Kings, Priests and Prophets

David of the tribe of Yehudah was the first King to be anointed with the *Shemen haMishchah*, and this one anointment would suffice for his male lineage forever, except when their throne was in dispute. Shlomo was anointed in haste at age twelve to secure his throne from Adoniya, who challenged his rule. His anointment was performed by the Prophet Natan, David's most trusted assistant. Likewise Yoash was anointed when his throne was in dispute by Atalia, and in the same way the Kingdom of Yehoahaz was secured from Yehoyakim.

Only the kings of the Davidic dynasty passed the kingdom from father to son, and they were exclusively commanded to use the original anointing oil of Moses. The oldest son would always be first in line to inherit the kingdom, including all of the holdings of Israel forever. Davidic kings were anointed only in Jerusalem, which was forbidden to Kings of any other lineage. Kings of another lineage were also not permitted to pass the throne down to their descendents. They were anointed only with *Shemen Afarsimon*, made from the same Judaic balsam that was used to produce the Temple incense. Since there were no Kings of the Davidic dynasty during the Second Temple period, the *Shemen haMishchah* was not employed, or even available for use. Most likely the jug that was hidden away in the final days of Solomon's Temple remained buried throughout the time of the Second Temple.

The young son of a king of the Davidic dynasty would need to wait until he was deemed old enough to inherit the kingdom, which was retained for him. It was required however that the son equal his father in wisdom and awe of the Holy One. If he was God-fearing but did not have wisdom, the elders would teach him; but if he was not God-fearing, he would not be worthy to inherit the kingdom from his father. Only a king who would keep all of God's commandments and fight God's battles was acceptable. All of David's sons were fit to inherit, and we learn that his kingdom and lineage will be restored to us in the future. The ultimate realization of this is the teaching that King Messiah will be a direct descendent of David. Since we learn that he will be anointed with the *Shemen haMichchah*, perhaps this indicates that his inheritance of David's kingdom will at first be in dispute.

A king must be anointed and crowned by a prophet, near a spring of living waters, by smearing the oil around his head like a crown. The living waters were a symbol that his reign should endure for many years. The anointment ceremony was repeated for a total of seven days, and always performed during the daytime.[9]

According to the Gemara,[10] a *Cohen Gadol* - High Priest - was anointed by making a Greek letter "*Kaf*" with the anointing oil, which is like the shape of an "X." The oil would be placed on the forehead, beginning with his eyebrows, and spread diagonally upwards. Other sources say that a Hebrew letter *Kaf* (for *Cohen* - priest) was used. In the Second Temple period there were approximately three hundred High Priests. A unique method of appointment was devised for all of them, as the *Shemen haMishchah* was apparently not available. During his initiation period, each High Priest would dress in eight items of special clothing commanded by the Torah, the *Bigdei Kodesh* - Holy Garments - purchased by the Temple treasury. Ceremoniously dressing in this distinctive clothing for seven days took the place of the anointment with oil.

The *Cohen Milchama* – Priest of War – was also anointed with the *Shemen haMishchah*.[11] He was responsible for leading Israel into battle, and his anointment for war would ensure that he would always bring victory to the nation by the hand of God, through his merit and righteousness. When approaching the battlefield, the *Cohen Milchama* would stand on a hill above his legions and proclaim: "Listen Israel, today you are about to wage war against your enemies. Do not be faint-hearted, do not be afraid, do not panic, and do not break ranks before them. God your Lord is the one who is going (to the battle) with you. He will fight for you against your enemies, and he will deliver you." His priestly assistants then spoke, dismissing and sending home all of those who had built a new house but not yet dwelt in it, planted a vineyard but not yet harvested it, or betrothed a woman but not yet consummated the marriage. The assistants then sent home all the faint-hearted, "rather than have his cowardliness demoralize his brethren."[12]

It is generally accepted in the mystery schools that the chief prophet of each generation was anointed by his predecessor. Rationalist and Kabbalistic Rabbis differ on this point. Rationalists say that prophets were only figuratively anointed, while priests and kings were literally anointed (with oil). Kabbalists say all three were literally anointed. Others say the earlier prophets were anointed as seer-priests, and formed prophecy schools. The "sons" of the prophets are the initiated members of these schools or mystery/prophecy guilds, the heads of which were anointed in each generation. The later prophets were solo figures answering God's call and were figuratively anointed, like Isaiah, by fire on the lips.[13]

There is evidence in Scripture that the chief prophet was anointed, when Elijah the Prophet is commanded by God to anoint Elisha as his successor, and also anoint Chaza'el as King of Aram; and Yehu ben Nimshi as King of Israel.[14] Elijah dies before he can carry out these tasks, and Elisha must complete them. Elisha sends his disciple (who Rashi identifies as Jonah) to anoint Yehu ben Nimshi.[15] One interesting question is what oil he used for the anointing. And what oil was used to anoint the King of Aram, also done by Hebrew prophets? Apparently neither Elijah nor Elisha nor Jonah went to the priests in Jerusalem to obtain the anointing oil of Moses to anoint the kings."[16]

Messiah: the Ultimate Anointment

Our Talmudic sages did not have a unified tradition of knowledge regarding the Messianic Age, and could only come to their conclusions by interpreting various Biblical passages. As a result, we find many opinions regarding these matters. The Messiah or "Anointed one" will be a direct descendent of King David who will restore his kingdom to its original state. He will also be a king who will rebuild the Temple and gather all the Jewish people together, no matter where they are scattered. Soon after that, the sacrifices, the Sabbatical – *Shemita*, and the Jubilee – *Yovel* - years will be restored, allowing us to observe all of the commandments of the Torah as in the days of old.

According to the "Principles of Maimonides,"[17] the Messiah will not need to perform miracles, will not necessarily change the course of nature nor bring the dead back to life. The Messiah will not alter the written Torah, which will remain the same forever. Just before the Messiah arrives, the Prophet Elijah will appear before the *Sanhedrin* – the Supreme Court of 71 righteous men, which will be re-established in Jerusalem. He will then be formally appointed by the Court[18] to anoint the Messiah with the holy anointing oil of Moses.[19]

The Torah promises, "God will restore your fortunes, have mercy on you, and gather you from all the countries where He has scattered you. If He were to banish you to the ends of the heavens you will be gathered in from there. The Lord your God will bring you to the land where your fathers dwelt. You will dwell there again, and He will make you even more prosperous and numerous than your fathers."[20] This passage includes the key predictions by the prophets regarding the people and land of Israel, and the Messiah.

We may assume that an individual is the Messiah if he fulfills the following conditions: He must be a king immersed in the Torah and its commandments, like David his ancestor. He must follow both our written and oral tradition, lead all Jews back to the Torah, strengthen the observance of its laws, and fight God's battles. If he does this successfully, and then rebuilds the Temple on its original site and gathers all of the dispersed Jews, then we may be certain that he is the Messiah. He will then bring the entire world to perfection, and inspire all people throughout the world to serve God in unity. It has been predicted, "I will then give all peoples a pure tongue that they may call in the name of God and all serve Him in one manner."[21] Everyone will keep the seven Noahide Laws; however, the ways of the world and the laws of nature will not change in the Messianic age. All nations will turn to holiness, and will no longer steal or oppress. They will enjoy only that which they have honestly attained, together with Israel.

Most scholars believe that the Messianic Age will begin with the war of Gog and Magog. Before this war, a prophet will arise to rectify the Jews and prepare their hearts: "Behold, I will send you Elijah the Prophet - *Eliahu HaNavi* - before the coming of the great and awesome day of God. He will turn the hearts of the fathers to the children, and the hearts of the children to their fathers."[22] From this we learn that the main task of Elijah will be to bring peace to the world. Other sages agree that Elijah will appear just before the Messiah, but they say that this will occur *after* the war of Gog and Magog. These teachings were purposely left ambiguous by our Prophets, and no one really knows exactly what will happen until the time arrives.

In the Messianic age, there will be neither war nor famine. Jealousy and competition will cease to exist, all good things will be most plentiful, and all sorts of delicacies will be common. The main pursuit of humanity will be to know the Holy One. The Jewish people will become great sages, know many hidden things, and achieve the greatest understanding of God possible for a mortal human being. As the Prophet Isaiah predicted, "The earth shall be full of the knowledge of God, as the waters cover the sea."[23]

The Messiah represents the pinnacle of spirituality, and the greatest consciousness any human being is capable of achieving in this world. A person at this exalted level is the ultimate expression of **fragrance** – both in personal emanation and receptivity. These two attributes are actually one: *emanating the most beautiful body scent is simply the "flip side" of having perfect fragrance perception.* The Messiah will emanate a heavenly personal scent reminiscent of the Temple incense and the Garden of Eden. At the same time, the Messiah will smell and thereby know all things, as he "will experience fragrance with the fear of God."[24] Our Rabbis have interpreted this to mean that through his remarkable sense of smell, the Messiah will be able to "smell the truth,"[25] to "sniff out" everyone's true character, and thus judge every person completely, fairly and accurately.

Since our Rabbis declare that our sense of smell is the most elevated aspect of our being, and our only sense that is still potentially as pure and holy today as it was in the Garden of Eden, we learn that it is our one true pathway back to the Garden. The Messiah - and each of us - must follow our noses to discern the truth and render judgment along our journey home. As scent is the primary vehicle of our enlightened super-consciousness, a person with reasonably good fragrance perception can smell and correctly identify his true aromatic medicines, his fragrant allies descended from the Garden, similar to the way that the Messiah will smell and know all things.

The Zohar speaks of the Messiah not only as being *initiated* by the anointing oil, but also as actually *being a physical embodiment* of the anointing oil, drawn from the main river flowing from the Garden of Eden. The implication is that the Messiah embodies the purpose of the anointing oil. He will radiate the fragrance and soul-essence of the Garden of Eden, as a model of the unified perfected soul of humanity.[16] His goal will be to inspire us all to rebuild our outer (and inner) Temple. In doing so, he will restore the beauty and exalted fragrance of the Garden of Eden to our environment, and elevate our consciousness to the bliss we enjoyed before we were expelled. Our mission to rebuild the outer and inner Temple will be achieved through self-sacrifice and devotion to the Holy One, at a level of moral and spiritual purification that will prepare the way for the redemption of the world under the enlightened and watchful guidance of the Messiah. As we return to the Garden, we will all finally merge into one heavenly fragrance, identical to the aroma of paradise and the scent of the Temple incense.

Personal Anointment

Each of our five senses is connected to an inner aspect of our being. Our sense of smell is deeply connected to our emotional state, and our various emotional states give off specific fragrances. This is the aromatic chemistry of our body scent, which becomes quite beautiful and attractive when we are in an overall state of good health. The most delightfully fragrant emanations are generated when the emotions are free of personality complexes and self-absorption. In short, *the more a person lets go of their ego and hang-ups, the more aromatically beautiful they will be*. The ego in surrender gives off the fragrance of a sweet perfume[26] and ultimately, the very fragrance of the holy Temple incense and paradise. The teachings regarding the Messiah demonstrate that having perfect fragrance perception and judgment ability is actually the "flip side" of being in perfect health. The Messiah will serve as a role model for all of us to reach this level.

While the use of the anointing oil as "God's perfume" was severely restricted, it served as a model and inspiration to everyone. The concept of anointment became increasingly widespread, and the practice of anointing oneself with aromatic oils was enjoyed by the general population. To "anoint" took on several different meanings. The most obvious, parallel to the use of the anointing oil, is the application of fragrant oils directly on the skin as a fragrant perfume that uplifts the soul, and has a pleasant aromatic effect on the body. This is still the basis of natural perfumery today, as presented in chapter 10. Another approach that was often used was to "anoint" the air with oil lamps and personal incense burners. Scented oils were also used to massage the body, or in a bath.

These are the ancient roots of our modern day forms of aromatherapy. Abundant information has emerged from many cultures regarding the properties and usage of hundreds of botanicals and their essential oils. While the anointing oil was an aromatic "skeleton key" that was precisely the right formulation for the kings and High Priests of Israel, the common person also needs his own personal remedy to support and complement his health. Natural essential oils have become increasingly available to meet this need, as the most concentrated, potent and sophisticated form of botanical medicine.

Anointing God: Blessings on Fragrances

Making a blessing is a mystical experience. It connects us with divine energetic pathways that empower us to fully enjoy the life-force pleasures of this world. Blessings transform the joy derived from the material world, and uplift the holy sparks back to their Source. The Talmud derives from the verse "every Soul praises God"[27] that it is fitting to make a blessing on a naturally-occurring substance which gives pleasure to the soul. This verse from Psalms establishes the importance of making blessings on fragrances, even on an enjoyable wisp of fragrance floating through the air, as fragrance delights the soul. There are five blessings for the fragrances of various plants, which closely correspond with five major blessings recited before eating different types of food.

Eating food also requires an "after-blessing," giving thanks to the Holy One at the conclusion of the meal. However, in contrast to food which nourishes the body for a limited "shelf-life," there is no after blessing for fragrances, since fragrance nourishes the Soul that is eternal. Similarly, no blessing of the season – *Shehecheyanu* – is said the first time a new fragrance is experienced in the new year, as the eternal nature of the soul is timeless.

The Hebrew calendar month of Nisan, which always comes in the spring, is the time of year for the renewal of fragrance in the world. The festival of Passover is celebrated on the 15th of Nisan, on the full moon. In the days of the Temple we began to offer only the fresh, newly-made batch of Temple incense starting on the first day of Nisan, when all the beautiful fragrances of nature come back to life, and begin emanating their heavenly scent from the vast multitude of aromatic trees, flowers and plants of creation.

In general we always make a blessing *before* smelling a pleasant fragrance or eating any type of food, as our Torah teaches us to bless the Holy One before we receive joy and sustenance in this world. However, it is important to test an *unfamiliar* fragrance first, *before* making a blessing, because a fragrance blessing is only permitted when the soul receives enjoyment. If you do not know whether or not the smell is pleasant, or how strong a fragrance is, or even whether or not your sense of smell is keen enough to enjoy the fragrance properly, as a trial you should smell it first without a blessing. When it becomes clear that the aroma is enjoyable to you, and that your soul will derive pleasure from the scent, the appropriate blessing should be recited just before smelling it carefully a second time and fully enjoying it.[28]

When more than one fragrant item is before us, we give priority to our personal preference and bless that item first. If a person has two flowers or two fragrant oils, he should first bless and enjoy his favorite. The "higher level" and more specific fragrance blessings take priority, whenever appropriate. With foods and fragrances, it is always preferable to recite the highest level of blessing possible, rather than just the general blessing, to further uplift and strengthen the divine connection. If one has a number of fragrant items before him that are all of the same category, only one blessing is recited. Below is a chart of the five levels of food and fragrance blessings. Note the correspondences between food and fragrance sources in each category:

Food Blessings	Made over	Fragrance Blessing	Made over
Hamotzi lechem min haAretz	Bread	***Boray Shemen Arev***	Balsam grown in Israel
Boray pri haGafen	Wine and Grape Juice	***Hanoten rayach tov b'payrot***	Fragrances from Citrus Fruits
Boray pri haEtz	Tree foods	***Boray atzay v'samim***	Trees, Perennial Fragrances
Boray pri Adama	Vegetables	***Boray isvay v'samim***	Grasses, Annual Fragrances
Shehakol nehiyeh b'divoroh	General Food Blessing	***Boray minay v'samim***	General Fragrance Blessing

The loftiest fragrance blessing of all, *Boray Shemen Arev* – "He who creates pleasing oil" - may only be recited on the aromatic derivatives of one species of tree, grown in a special location: the extremely rare Judaic balsam of Gilead, *Commiphora opobalsamum*. This blessing can only be made when the tree was cultivated in Israel, and as a result this blessing has not been recited for over 1,500 years. Judaic balsam trees still exist today, but only in the regions of Mecca and Medina, Saudi Arabia. These rare trees are carefully guarded and not exported. Over the fragrance of the much more common Peru balsam, which grows abundantly in Central America, we recite the blessing on perennial tree fragrances.

The blessing on fragrances from fruits, *Hanoten rayach tov b'payrot* – "He who gives fruit a good scent" - is said on the whole fruit and on the Essential oil extracted from the skin. On fruit peels alone, when they have already been separated from the fruit, the general blessing is said. The blessing for trees, *Boray atzay v'samim* – "He who creates aromatic trees" – is said over perennial plants whose leaves grown from branches rather than straight out of the ground. Blessings made on grasses, *Boray isvay v'samim* – "He who creates aromatic plants" are said over annual plants that must be seasonally cultivated, or which fully regenerate themselves each year, or whose leaves come straight out of the ground.

When a fragrance is pulverized, a distilled essential oil, or placed into a carrier vegetable oil, the blessing remains the same as the one recited on the original plant material before it was processed. When there is any doubt, recite the general fragrance blessing *Boray minay v'samim* – "He who creates a variety of spices/perfumes" - which is always acceptable on any pleasant natural fragrance. This general blessing is also said over a group of fragrances of different categories, or when a particular fragrance falls into different categories.

No blessing is said over chemical "perfumes" or any other synthetic fragrance, as they are very unhealthy substances and certainly not a gift of nature. No blessing is said on fragrances that have an unpleasant or neutral odor, or which are too strong or too weak to give enjoyment to the soul. A blessing may be recited on a pleasant and recognizable aroma in the air, but no blessing is said on the fragrance of a neighbor's freshly baked bread during Passover. On the Sabbath, the sages forbid smelling and blessing a fragrant fruit that is still growing on a tree, as it might lead one to pick and enjoy that fruit. However, on the Sabbath smelling and blessing a fragrant flower that is still growing is fully permitted. So, we can always take time to smell (and bless) the Roses!

Chapter 5

The Recovery of the Lost Ark of the Covenant

Almost everyone is familiar with Steven Spielberg's blockbuster movie, "Raiders of the Lost Ark," in which the hero Indiana Jones searches for the Ark of the Covenant. This is a fictional movie, yet the screenplay is mysteriously connected to the amazing *true story* of the great archaeologist and Biblical scholar Dr. Vendyl Jones. This same adventurous, loveable and not so fictitious character was also portrayed in several other Spielberg films.

Perhaps an even more remarkable man in real life than the hero portrayed in the movies, Vendyl Miller Jones (b. May 29, 1930 in Sudan, Texas) was once a Christian pastor who left his post to become the worldwide leader of the growing Noahide movement. His followers are God-fearing non-Jews who observe the seven Noahide Laws, which are based on truth, justice, peaceful co-existence and are relevant to all of humanity. The enigmatic explorer and teacher published a book in 1959 predicting the precise outbreak of the Six Day War. Based on his analyses of events during the Exodus from Egypt and up until the First Temple period, he transposed the same timeline onto our current Third Temple period - an era which began with the foundation of the Jewish State in the Land of Israel in 1948. The Patriarch Abraham also came to Israel in the year 1948 on the *Hebrew* calendar, which was nearly four thousand years ago. Vendyl says that when we apply Biblical analyses to modern times, this can alert us to important upcoming global events - true modern adventures which will ultimately "turn the world right-side-up!"

Dr. Jones, who has a photographic memory, has been active for the past forty years in a very dedicated search for the *real* Ark of the Covenant, as well as many other amazing and priceless treasures of the Temple, sacred vessels which were covertly put into long-term storage about 2,600 years ago. These unique and irreplaceable items were hidden away by the Prophet Jeremiah and his disciples, seven years before the destruction of the First Temple of Solomon.[1] As the Talmud explains, Jeremiah foresaw prophetically that the exile was imminent, and certain holy implements had to be secured for future generations who would need them in the days of the Messiah and the Third Temple. Jeremiah thus directed King Josiah to hide the Ark of the Covenant, along with many of the other precious Temple vessels and treasures. All of these sacred items, together with enormous quantities of gold and silver, appear to all be hidden in one long-secret underground cavern area - which Vendyl Jones is convinced that he has recently located.

Historically, we know that just as Jeremiah had prophesized, King Nebuchadnezzar of Babylon sent his armies on a mission to conquer Jerusalem. These forces finally overran the surrounding walls, sacked the Holy City, destroyed the Temple and carried the Jewish population off into exile. The invaders also carried away with them the holy vessels that they found in the Temple, but apparently they never discovered the hidden cache of the original Temple treasures - the holy articles that had been in use in the Tabernacle and Temple services, from the time of the revelation at Mt. Sinai, until just prior to the Babylonian exile. These items, including the Ark, remain well hidden today.

According to the studies and explorations of Dr. Jones, the original treasures of the Temple, such as the Ark of the Covenant, were never actually captured or discovered. The reason why this is true is because several years preceding the destruction of the Temple, replicas were secretly made to replace most of the original vessels, and all of the genuine items were then safely hidden away. The invading Babylonian army captured and carried away only these replicas. Also, the original Temple treasures crafted by Betzalel were not buried in the area of the Temple Mount as is commonly believed, as that would have soon led to their capture by the conquering army. King Solomon in his great wisdom, with the assistance of the prophets, foresaw a time when his Temple would be under attack, completely surrounded by enemy forces, and destroyed. Thus they realized that an emergency escape route must be designed and included in the construction of the Temple, which would provide for the safe evacuation of the Temple treasures and personnel under these dire circumstances. This led to a highly secretive decision to build a holding chamber area underneath the Temple for temporary storage, and dig a long connecting passageway to a distant safe escape area. This long-secret information is still not widely known today, even by many of our most respected religious authorities.

For many years, Dr. Jones has had remarkable success in analyzing a unique and amazing old treasure map, produced about 2,600 years ago. The data that has emerged has led his team to recover a juglet of the original anointing oil of Moses in 1988; a huge cache of Temple incense in 1992; and to pinpoint in 1995 the exact site of the early encampment of Gilgal. These discoveries resulted from a careful decoding of a unique metallic document, known as the **Copper Scroll**, which was personally dictated by the prophet Jeremiah. His words were transcribed in great haste onto the back of the copper plate, in reverse script, by five men alternately working with a hammer and stylus.

The future recovery of the legendary Ark of the Covenant, also being tracked through advanced deciphering of this very document, may soon be Vendyl's crowning achievement. The Talmud mentions that the Ark and the other holy vessels of Solomon's Temple were at first *temporarily* hidden "in a secret vault underneath the Temple Mount." Dr. Jones has revealed that this storage area was connected to a long underground tunnel, which stretched eastward in descending elevation for a distance of 18 miles. The other end of this passageway reaches the Valley of Achor by the Dead Sea, alongside an area where a complex of hidden underground chambers known as the "Cave of the Column" is located. According to Dr. Jones, this is the long hidden location of the Temple treasures to this day.

About 50 years before the destruction of Solomon's Temple and the Babylonian Exile, Josiah, the last righteous King of Judea, ascended the throne at the tender age of 8. By the 18th year of his reign, King Josiah had ordered sweeping religious reforms, as well as extensive repairs to the Temple building. During these renovations, a rare Torah scroll personally written by Moses was discovered, hidden under the stones in the floor of the Temple. Upon inspection, it was found that this scroll was wound to intentionally display certain verses in the 28th Chapter of Deuteronomy, which read as follows:

> "God will bring you and your elected king to a nation unknown to you and your fathers, and there you will serve idolaters who worship wood and stone. You will be an object of horror... You will bring much seed out to the field, but the locusts will devour (the crop)... you will plant vineyards and work hard, but the worms will eat (the grapes)... you will have olive trees in all of your territories, but the olives will drop off (before rip-

> ening)... you will have sons and daughters, but they will not remain yours, since they will be taken into captivity... the alien among you will rise higher and higher over you, while you will descend lower and lower... all of these curses will thus have come upon you... and all because you did not obey God your Lord, and (did not) keep the commandments and decrees that He prescribed to you. (These curses) will be a sign and a proof to you and your children forever."[2]

Jeremiah and King Josiah reacted to the discovery of this Torah scroll, and its bookmarked place, as an ominous sign that Jerusalem and the Temple would soon fall into enemy hands, and the people of Israel taken into captivity. They ordered that substitute Temple vessels be constructed immediately to replace the original vessels in use, although no replacement was ever constructed for the Ark of the Covenant, as it was considered too holy to replicate. Jeremiah then organized the removal of the Ark and many other original vessels to the secret underground storage area beneath the Temple Mount, which had been prepared by King Solomon when the Temple was constructed. The transfer of the vessels was recorded by Jeremiah's companion, Shimur HaLevi, who also made a complete inventory of all that was stored away. This special underground-chamber aspect of the Temple design is mentioned in Scripture [Kings II], but according to rabbinic tradition, the long passageway connecting the underground chamber to the Dead Sea area was known only to certain priests and kings of Israel. This greatest secret of the Temple design was never directly recorded or publicly revealed, although it is covertly referred to in Kings II in describing the escape from the Temple of King Zedekiah.[3]

In the Hebrew calendar year 3303 the original vessels were removed from the Temple to the underground storage area, and the replicas were immediately put into place. This was done in haste to keep the Temple services functioning daily, and also to hide the fact that the original treasures had been secretly stored underneath the Temple Mount. The hidden items included the Ark of the Covenant, the desert Tabernacle, the Temple incense altar, the golden Menorah, most of the anointing oil prepared by Moses, the *Kelal* vessel containing the ashes of the red heifer, the staff of Aaron, the breastplate, the vestments of the High Priest, the rod, and the pot of manna, among many other priceless treasures including vast amounts of gold and silver from the Temple treasury.[4]

In the year 3316, King Josiah died in battle defending the Judaic kingdom against Pharaoh Necho II, and Judea became a vassal to Egypt. Soon afterwards, Nebuchadnezzar of Babylon expanded his campaign to plunder the land of Israel and take control of Jerusalem. As the Babylonian armies intensified their effort to conquer the Holy Land, in the year 3331 Jeremiah and five of his colleagues (Shimur Ha-Levi, Zedekiyahu, Yizkiyahu, Haggai the Prophet and Zachariah, the son of Ido the Prophet), along with three hundred priests, and Levites "without number," covertly performed the sacred mission of moving the Temple treasures to their final safety. All of the vessels were moved out of the storage area underneath the Temple Mount, and transported underground through the 18-mile passageway to their current resting place in the chambers of the "Cave of the Column" complex near the Dead Sea, where they remain securely concealed today.

Finally in the year 3338, the Babylonians conquered Jerusalem and breached the walls of the Temple. King Zedekiah, together with a small entourage, fled the Temple to avoid capture. No doubt to protect the whereabouts of the Temple treasures, no specific reference to a tunnel is mentioned in scripture. However, from a close study of the language of the Second Book of Kings, it is evident that their escape was made through the long underground passageway leading to the Dead Sea:

> "And the City [Jerusalem] was besieged until the eleventh year of King Zedekiyahu. And on the ninth day of the fourth month the famine prevailed in the City, and there was no bread for the people of the land. And a breach was made in the City, and all the men of war fled by night *by the way of the Gate between the two walls*, which is by the king's garden. (Now the *Kasdim* - Babylonian army - were against the City round about), and they (the king's entourage) went in the direction of the *Arava* (desert plains). And the army of the *Kasdim* pursued after the king, and overtook him in the plains of Jericho, and all of (the king's) armies were scattered from him."[5]

Since the Babylonian army had *completely surrounded* Jerusalem and the Temple, a secret underground passage was the *only* possible escape route. The need for this emergency exit for those who were trapped within the Temple, as well as for the previous evacuation of the Temple treasures, must have been envisioned by the contractor, King Solomon. He was well aware of a series of prophetic revelations, beginning long before the Temple was constructed, forecasting the ultimate destruction of Jerusalem. Unfortunately, in spite of their brilliant escape, King Zedekiah and his group were soon captured by Babylonian soldiers who were hunting in the plains of Jericho near the Dead Sea. The soldiers had chased a deer into a cave, and came upon the royal escapees entirely by surprise.

Yet the sacred treasures of the Temple remained safe and undiscovered, having been transported through this same tunnel seven years previously, and then carefully and fully concealed in underground chambers near the end of the tunnel, by the Valley of Achor. The area of the "gate between the two walls" tunnel entrance just underneath the Temple Mount, mentioned in Kings II, as well as sections of the tunnel itself, were explored by Vendyl Jones in 1967, just before all access to this area was sealed off by the Israeli authorities. This resulted after Jones had informed them that he had discovered several Arabs emerging from within the tunnel, in an area where enemy ammunition might be stored.

Immediately after the Temple treasures were concealed, scrolls and tablets were hastily produced by the assistants of Jeremiah, under his precise direction. Among these was the Copper Scroll, mentioned above. These documents were prepared in order to preserve a long-term record of crucial information concerning the hidden Temple treasures. The details that were recorded included pinpointing their exact hiding places, references to specific identifying marks, and instructions on how to renew and re-enlist each holy vessel into service, to reinstitute the various Temple ceremonies. The documents were then also hidden away by these same men.

At a later time during the Babylonian Exile, some of this information was also preserved in writings that were included in early Talmudic literature. Due to its secretive nature, most of these passages were subsequently removed from later editions of the Talmud, although some early records have survived. However, none of these Talmudic writings (nor any other known ancient writings) included the crucial information hammered onto the Copper Scroll, which cryptically encodes the exact location where the Ark of the Covenant and the other holy vessels are hidden. Revealing the geographical co-ordinates of the hidden treasures in 64 specific locations is the main focus of this document. These precious secrets were closely guarded and carefully preserved, passed down through time only on this one copper plate, hidden in a secret chamber near the Dead Sea. This information was only intended to be revealed at the "End of Days," and then only to those who could solve the puzzle of how to read and interpret the Copper Scroll correctly.

There were all together *four* individual documents produced by Jeremiah and his men, that relate to and describe the hidden treasures of the Temple. They were written and concealed shortly after the holy vessels were hidden. These four artifacts are the fragments of an ancient map, intended to help us locate and identify these treasures, and put them back into use in the days of the Third Temple:

a. The **Copper Scroll** is a plaque made of the purest copper, seven feet wide, which contains a list of the concealed holy treasures from the First Temple, and the exact locations where they were hidden, just before the Babylonian conquest. It has been engraved in reverse writing from the back side to produce raised Hebrew letters on the surface, and could not be deciphered without knowledge of Rabbinical vocabulary and literature. Some of the text is clearly readable, but in other areas it is a jumble of half-sentences, dead ends and squiggle marks that defied interpretation by world-class graphologists for nearly 40 years. During this time, it was considered by most archaeologists to be a forgery, or "the work of a madman." Jones discovered that the Scroll revealed key secrets when read in a diagonal order and other very unusual ways. The Copper Scroll was discovered in two rolled segments, stacked one on top of the other, in cave #3 at Qumran on March 20, 1952, very close to the area where the Dead Sea Scrolls were found four years earlier. To open it for study, it was carefully sliced into 23 sections. Today it remains the property of the Jordanian government, and is currently on public display in the central historical museum of Amman, Jordan.

b. The **Silver Scroll** contains an inventory list, and an explanation of all that was hidden, with private inventory marks corresponding to marks that are engraved on each item. This Scroll remains undiscovered to this day. Jones believes that it is hidden together with the *Kelal* (a vessel containing the ashes of the red heifer, necessary for ritual purification in order to reinstitute the Temple services), very close to the location of the Ark of the Covenant, in the Cave of the Column complex at Qumran.

c. Two **Marble Tablets** - *Massaket Kelim* - contain verses describing the treasures and how they were hidden. The same verses were inscribed in early versions of the codified Talmud, but were later removed from the written text to guard this information. The wording on the Tablets begins: "These are the words of Shimur HaLevi, the servant of God, in the year 3331 of Adam." The remainder of the text, without this introduction, also appears in the Naftaly Hertz book "*Emek HaMelech*," mentioned above. The Tablets were apparently first hidden at Mt. Carmel, and finally discovered over 2,500 years later in 1952 in the basement storage vault of a museum in Beirut, Lebanon. They later vanished again. Vendyl Jones believes that a wealthy Jewish family in Syria obtained them, and has them in safekeeping.

d. An **Ibex Scroll** of goat skin, also known as "the Temple Scroll." This manuscript makes reference to the Copper Scroll, and contains verses of detailed instructions on how to re-institute the Temple services, once the hidden vessels have been recovered. It was written in the first person, leading some scholars to believe that these chapters were transmitted directly by God to Moses. These are the same uncodified verses found in the Marble Tablets and in *Emek HaMelech*. The Ibex Scroll was discovered in 1963 in a cave at Qumran near the Copper Scroll cave, by the same Bedouin who found the Dead Sea Scrolls in 1947. Today it is housed in the Israel Museum, although the scroll is no longer on public display as exposure to light was causing deterioration.

The Copper Scroll includes exact information on the secret hidden location of the Ark of the Covenant and the other Holy Vessels, *which were never recovered for use during the days of the Second Temple*, except a cache of Temple incense which was buried separately. This is remarkable, since the locations of the secret hiding places of the Ark and vessels were well known to Haggai, Zachariah (the last of the later Prophets), and others who were present at the destruction of the First Temple, and returned to Jerusalem for the rebuilding and dedication of the Second Temple 70 years later. Those who knew the hidden location of the treasures very intentionally did not make use of this information in order to recover these items upon their return. They could clearly see that the Second Temple would never compare to the greatness of Solomon's Temple. Only the Third Temple period was foreseen as the time when the treasures would be needed in the exalted "Days of Messiah," as described in the text of the Marble Tablets and the Ibex Scroll.

Early Talmudic writings which include excerpts from some of these original documents, except for the Copper Scroll, have occasionally resurfaced. One obscure mystical text, *Emek HaMelech* ("Valley of the King"), published in Amsterdam in 1648, is a reprinting of a very rare, early Talmudic discourse which was later hidden away. The author of this text, Rabbi Naftali Hertz, was a very holy and prominent Talmudic scholar, whose knowledge of both the written and oral Torah was superb. He was in the lineage of a most illustrious group of Rabbis, including famous Kabbalist Rabbi Yitzhak Luria, and Rabbi Yosef Cairo, the author of the *Shulchan Aruch* - Code of Jewish Law.

Rabbi Hertz cites as his source for the passages in his text an ancient *Tosephta* - forgotten addition - to the Talmud, related to Mishnah 3 in *Kelim* - vessels. However, any reference to the Temple vessels was completely removed from more modern editions of this same *Tosephta*. Hertz obviously had access to a rare ancient manuscript, and perhaps it was passed down to him by one of his illustrious ancestors.

Emek Hamelech clearly demonstrates the accurate and unbroken transmission of secret knowledge through written records, revealing part of the information that was hidden away on documents of parchment and stone by Jeremiah and his men, more than two thousand years before this publication emerged. Certain sections of the Talmudic wording in the text closely match the inscriptions on the Marble Tablets and the Ibex Scroll, which were finally recovered more than three hundred years *after* the text was published. A complete translation of this remarkable text is presented at the end of this Chapter.

Through a painstaking study of the Copper Scroll over many years, his patience and fortitude finally paid off in April 1988 when Vendyl

Jones and his team of B'nai Noach volunteers located an ancient juglet of thick oil, which was found in the vicinity of the Copper Scroll cave. Intensive testing by the Pharmaceutical Department of Hebrew University concluded that the substance inside this vessel was indeed the genuine anointing oil of Moses. This is the third juglet put to use of the original twenty-four that Moses prepared, the vessel that had been employed for over 1,000 years to anoint kings and priests of Israel. Since - as far as we know - the anointing oil was not used at all during the Second Temple period, it is assumed that this juglet was hidden in the final days of the First Temple, close to the time when over 400 Kg of Temple incense was buried.

This amazing find was a landmark discovery in another way, as it was the very first time that an item was actually located by deciphering a section of the Copper Scroll. Now the authenticity of this document seemed indisputable. Dozens of major networks and news sources carried the story worldwide. Rabbi Menachem Burstein, the foremost authority on the botany and chemistry of Temple artifacts, affirmed that the discovery was an early sign that we were rapidly moving towards the restoration of the Holy Temple. This juglet is on display at the Israel Museum in Jerusalem.

To this day, the remaining twenty one juglets of anointing oil are still hidden away, stored inside of the Ark of the Covenant. Worlds beyond being a simple storage chest, the Ark apparently has the unique power to indefinitely preserve the life-force of the items stored inside of it. Remarkably, it seems to function as an energetic "deep freezer." This would explain how most of the anointing oil - which can never be reproduced – will stay fresh until the "End of Days," when it will be needed to anoint the Messiah. We can assume that the anointing oil has always been safely stored inside of the Ark, since the time when it was first produced by Moses. This includes over 1,000 years of storage before the Ark was hidden away by Jeremiah.

Since it is a commandment of the Torah for all of the people of Israel to insure that the anointing oil is used according to the divine instructions given to Moses, any representative of our people who is on a quest that would allow us to fulfill our holy work deserves our full support. At a meeting with the Lubavitcher Rebbe z"l on July 1, 1990, the Rebbe said to Vendyl Jones: "You are doing the most important work in the world. Many people will try to make you stop what you are doing.

Many people will try to make you change what you are doing. Don't stop, and don't change what you are doing, and God will Bless you. God Bless you. God Bless you!"

About two years later in March 1992, near Qumran at the north-western corner of the Dead Sea, Jones and his team discovered an underground bedrock silo which contained over 900 lbs. of an aromatic red-brown powder. This treasure was also found in the same area as the Copper Scroll cave. The powder was later shown to be authentic ancient Temple incense. It had been sealed in an air-tight underground limestone chamber for long-term safekeeping, and hidden in a separate location apparently in the year 68 CE, two years before the destruction of the Second Temple. Temple incense was used throughout the Second Temple period. Yet the Copper Scroll, written nearly 500 years earlier, mysteriously revealed the location of this hiding place as well. How is this possible? This must have been the very same location that was previously used to hide incense at the end of the First Temple period. The location was found by excavating the mound highlighted by the mysterious "Blue Aura," an extraordinary lighting feature inside the cave mentioned on the first plate of the Copper Scroll. This was used as a descriptive landmark by those who hid the Temple treasures.

A chemical analysis of the red-brown material by Dr. Martin Antelman, a consultant to the Weitzman Institute, revealed that it contains at least nine of the spices of the Temple incense in a highly refined state, and perhaps as many as all eleven spices. Subsequently the pollens in the material were identified by Dr. Terry Hutter, a paleobotanist. This analysis also helped to determine exactly which spices were used to make the incense, a matter of great debate among top rabbinical scholars for centuries. I first met Vendyl Jones shortly after this chemical analysis of his discovered material was published, and the findings that he presented in his Report entitled "The Copper Scroll and the excavations at Qumran" allowed me to nearly complete my set of Temple incense oils.

There was great interest regarding whether or not this ancient Temple incense powder, nearly 2,000 years old, would still have any aromatic properties when burned. At the request of Israel's Chief Rabbis, a tiny sample of the red-brown material was carefully ignited with sulfuric acid in a laboratory experiment performed by Jones, as burning it with fire might violate the prohibition against personal use of the incense.

Those present reported that even though the mixture had been buried for so long, the resulting fragrance was "entrancingly beautiful and persistent, lingering for months afterwards."

Hidden together in the chamber with the incense, Jones found 3 to 4 lbs. of what appeared to be "Sodom salt" crystals in the form of chips or flakes, and about 4 cubic meters (25-30 lbs.) of "Karshina lye," which Vendyl says is actually the ash that collected underneath the outer Temple altar. A question was raised about why these materials were separate, but buried together with the spice mixture, rather than already incorporated during production. It is quite possible that these materials were necessary to complete the blend, and make it into finished incense. The spice mixture did not actually become genuine Temple incense *until all* of the ingredients were combined together as specified. In an unfinished form, the spice mixture was not subject to the same Jewish ritual requirements and restrictions as the finished Temple incense would be. This was a protection for all people who might come in contact with it, legitimately or otherwise, as very strong prohibitions forbid private use.

One might think that the Karshina lye was used to process the "*Tziporren*" spice separately, before it was included in the mixture. However, the fact that it is cited as a separate ingredient also might indicate that the entire amount specified was included as a final ingredient. Thus the bleaching process would be a result over time of the final incorporation of the Karshina lye with the entire mixture. Once it was added, a chemical reaction might begin to take place, transforming the mixture into a whole new substance. Like a fine wine, the incense would age, ever so slightly. After a certain calculated and observed amount of time, this bleaching process would terminate when the finished product was ready to be burned.

Similarly, the Sodom salt may have been a final added ingredient, due to the reaction it might cause over time. It is also possible that the Sodom salt itself was actually the mysterious "smoke-raising herb." In both the cases of the lye and the salt, had they been incorporated with the spice mixture before it was buried, the Ketoret might have become ruined by over-reaction during the long exile. Finally, seemingly in support of the above theory, the Chief Rabbis instructed Vendyl to carefully add the discovered lye and salt to the spice mixture before he ignited it in his experiment, which he did.

In 1994, our relentless explorer embarked upon a study together with the Israeli Petroleum, Geology and Geophysics Institute to use ground penetrating radar (GPR) technology onsite at the Cave of the Column. This equipment uses high frequency radio emissions together with computer analyses to examine the underlying bedrock and geological formations of any given area. The GPR survey conducted at the Cave of the Column confirmed the existence of the massive chamber described in the Copper Scroll. This reading was subsequently confirmed by electrical resistivity work in 1998, which carefully measured the underground cavity to be 25 feet high and 65 feet wide. Dr. Vendyl Jones believes that this is surely the ancient hiding place of the Ark of the Covenant and the long lost treasures of the Temple.

More recently, a prominent unnamed kabbalist has given a blessing to Dr. Jones to uncover the Holy Ark of the Covenant. The Ark is the resting place of the two tablets of the Ten Commandments, endowed to Moses and the Jewish people at Mt. Sinai. Throughout the many years of his quest, Jones has been in close contact with and under the guidance of the Chief Rabbis of Israel, Rabbi Adin Steinsaltz, and other illustrious rabbis and kabbalists. Extremely knowledgeable himself in Torah, Talmud and Kabbalistic sources dealing with holy Temple issues, Dr. Jones has now received permission from both known and hidden kabbalists to finally uncover the Lost Ark. He believes that this most amazing discovery in history is only a matter of time, as the Jewish prophecies regarding the greatly anticipated redemption are occurring right in front of our eyes.

At the time when the famous film was produced, Jones was far from pinpointing the location of the Ark, although he has come a long way since then. Continuing to decipher the text and precise layout of the Copper Scroll with the help of international graphology experts, Jones was convinced that he finally knew the exact location of the Ark of the Covenant.

When I recently asked Dr. Jones what he would do with the Ark once it has been excavated, he responded that at that point it would no longer be his responsibility, or in his realm of authority: "That will depend on the Chief Rabbis of Israel, and their key assistants such as Rabbi Steinsaltz." I then asked him if he had any idea about what they will do with it. His response was that he had suggested to Rabbi Steinsaltz that the Ark be moved immediately to Gilgal, the location of the first

Israelite encampment in the Land of Israel at the end of the Exodus. This is a location at the northern edge of the Dead Sea where the Ark rested for fourteen years, when first arriving in the Holy Land after crossing the Jordan River. *Dr. Jones himself identified that precise location* in 1994, also through a careful analyses of the Copper Scroll and the use of infrared thermal remote sensing equipment.

The Noahide leader believes that when these holy treasures are found, it will usher in a new period in Jewish history, leading to the building of the Third Temple, the Messianic Age and profound implications for world peace. But before the Temple can be rebuilt in Jerusalem, the Land of Israel and its people must be ritually purified and renewed. Since Israel had it first beginnings at Gilgal when we first entered the Land after the Exodus, the kingdom will once again be renewed at Gilgal. The state of Israel is passing through the same Biblical channels as the generation that first entered the Land from Egypt. "If history repeats itself, then history itself is prophecy. Israel is different from all other nations in a lot of ways, but more than anything else, Israel is the only nation whose history was written *before* it happened," he said.

Dr. Vendyl Jones believes that when the ashes of the red heifer, the desert Tabernacle and the Ark on the Covenant are found, they will be initially taken back to Gilgal, where the Priesthood will be ritually purified and where the kingdom will be spiritually and politically renewed in preparation for the rebuilding of the Third Temple in Jerusalem. The ancient desert Tabernacle, which includes the Ark, will remain in Gilgal until the day that God sends his messenger, whose right and responsibility it is to return the Ark of the Covenant to its final resting place on the Temple Mount in Jerusalem.

Aftermath

To get a good overview of the work and teachings of Vendyl Jones and what drove him, I suggest that you read Vendyl's self-penned memoir, "A Door of Hope: My Search for the Treasures of the Copper Scroll." It is published by Vendyl's close friend and disciple Jim Long of Lightcatcher Productions. In November 2011, an important message arrived from Jim with an update:

"Vendyl passed away following complications from throat cancer [on Dec. 27th, 2010]. Thanks to the care he received, his passing came with relative calm. The most notable aspect of his death is that, according to the Hebrew calendar, he shares the very same *yartzheit* [date of death] as the Rambam [Maimonides]. So, it's quite fitting that he was laid to rest in a region of Israel where many of Israel's great sages are also interred. Per his wishes, we buried him in a small Noachide cemetery adjacent to the Jewish cemetery on the outskirts of Migdol [in northern Israel by the Sea of Galilee].

"He has quite a legacy because of his efforts for Noachides. There is no particular person that has been designated as his immediate successor. That's because, thanks to him, there are so many of us doing what we can to spread the message of Torah and the [7 Noachide laws]. In fact, I'm convinced that he will be remembered for making people aware of the 7 Laws even more than anything else. It seems to me that [God] used Vendyl's archaeological work to spread the truth of Torah. After meeting him in 1993, I was often with him as he addressed rapt audiences who had filled lecture halls to hear [about] his exploits. Many didn't realize the lectures were laced with Torah teachings. Regarding his archaeological work, the only person that I know of who is both capable and motivated to carry it on is David Ben Avraham who possesses a real-world grasp of methods required to actually dig at the site [areas near the Dead Sea where Vendyl was exploring].

"As far as I know, [Vendyl] didn't tell anyone where he thought the Ark of the Covenant was located. In 2010, during his final visit to Israel, a small party (including myself) accompanied him to the Cave of the Column. His plan was to sink a small shaft near a specific rock that he'd marked on a previous visit. He would drop a 'lipstick cam' into that shaft. This device, as the name implies, resembles a small lipstick tube. It's a high resolution video camera with an on-board light source, connected to a video recorder. Due his failing memory, Vendyl couldn't locate the rock or even recall the exact place that he wanted to sink the shaft that would lead into a chamber holding [the] ancient treasures. It was not to be."

Jim Long

Lightcatcher Productions • www.lightcatcherprod.com

****

The following is an abridged translation of the introduction and the first 9 Chapters of the sacred text *Emek HaMelech*.[6] The original verses are from the period of the Babylonian Exile, first transmitted shortly after the First Temple was destroyed. This ancient Talmudic text was written down and published under the title *Emek HaMelech* in 1648 by Rabbi Naftali Hertz. His volume was recently republished in Hebrew.

"These documents (the four treasure maps) were written by five righteous men (under the command of Jeremiah): Shimur the Levite, Hizkiyah, Zidkiya, Chaggai the Prophet and Zechariah, son of Ido the Prophet. These men concealed the vessels of the Temple and treasures of Jerusalem, which will not be discovered until the day of the coming of the Messiah, son of David, speedily in our times, Amen, and so it will be.

Mishnah 1

"These are the vessels dedicated and concealed when the Temple was destroyed: The Tabernacle and the curtain, the holy Menorah, the Ark of Testimony, the golden forehead nameplate, the golden crown of Aaron the Priest, the Breastplate of Judgment, the silver trumpets, the Cherubim, the altar of burnt offerings, the curtain of the Communion Tent, the forks and the bread molds, the bread Table, the curtain of the Gate, the Copper Altar, the sacred garments of Aaron which were worn by the High Priest on the Day of Atonement, bells and pomegranates on the hem of the robe of the High Priest, the holy vessels that Moses made on Mt. Sinai by the command of the Holy One, the Staff, and the jar of Manna.

Mishnah 2

"These are the Holy vessels and the vessels of the Temple that were in Jerusalem and in every place (where the Tabernacle traveled). They were inscribed by Shimur HaLevi and his companions on a *Luach Nehoshet* - Copper Scroll, with all the vessels of the Holy of Holies that Shlomo son of David made. And together with Shimur were Hizkiyahu, Zidkiyah, Haggai the Prophet, and Zechariah, son of Berachiah, son of Ido the Prophet."

Mishnah 3

"These are the vessels that were buried in the ground: the locking rods, the pegs, the boards, the rings, the standing pillars of the courtyard. These are the vessels: 1,200,000 silver sacrificial basins - *Mizkarot*; 50,000 basins of fine gold; 600,000 (?) of fine gold, and 1,200,000 of silver. These five men inscribed these *Mishnayot* – verses - in Babylon together with the other prophets that were with them, including Ezra the Cohen, the scribe.

Mishnah 4

"Of the Levites, 130 were killed and 100 escaped with Shimur Ha-Levi and his companions. These men concealed 500,000 trays of fine gold, and 1,200,000 of silver; 500,000 bread molds of fine gold, and 1,200,000 of silver. On each of the molds there were 5 *Margaliot* - pearls? - and 2 precious gem stones. The value of each precious stone was 100 talents of gold, and the total value of all the *Margaliot* was 200,000 talents of gold. There were also 36 golden trumpets. All of these were hidden and concealed in a tower in the land of Babylon, in the great city called Baghdad. (There was also a 7-branched) Menorah of fine gold, (worth) 100,000 (talents), with 7 lamps on each (branch), 26 precious gem stones on each Menorah, each *Margalit* priceless, and between every gem stone, 200 (smaller) stones, also priceless.

Mishnah 5

"There were 77 tables of gold, and gold (hangings) from the walls of the Garden of Eden that was revealed to Shlomo. Their radiance was like the brilliance of the sun and the moon that shine above the world. And all the silver and gold that ever existed in the world, from the six days of Creation until the day that Zidkiyahu became king, did not equal the value of the gold that was overlaid on the Temple from within and from without. There is no end, no measure, no set amount, and no weighing of the gold that overlaid the Temple and the face of the Temple. All this, plus another 7,000 talents of gold, were brought and concealed in the *Segel Habar* (?) with precious stones with which the Temple was built, besides three rows of priceless stones, and one row of *Almugim* - sandalwood? - trees... David prepared all of these for the Great House (the Temple), for Shlomo, his son.

Mishnah 6

"The number of building stones was 36,000, the same as the number of gem stones. From all of these the Temple was built. There were also three-plus-one rows of *Almugim* trees, overlaid with fine gold and placed in the building. All those were hidden from Nebuchadnezzar by the fittest men of Israel. The *Almugim* shine like the brilliance of the firmament (sky).

Mishnah 7

"The counting of precious stones, *Margaliot* gems, silver and gold that King David dedicated to the great Temple was: 1,000,000 talents of silver, 100,000 talents of gold and trees made of "*Parvaim* gold" which bore fruit, 600,000 talents of fine gold from beneath the Tree of Life in the holy Garden. All these were revealed to Hilkiyah the scribe, who gave them into the safekeeping of the angel Shimshiel to guard until King David arises, to whom he will hand over the silver and gold, including the gold that Shlomo contributed, and the talents of gold and priceless precious stones. All these were concealed, hidden, and safeguarded from the army of the Chaldeans in a place called Borseef.

Mishnah 8

"There were seven golden curtains that contained 12,000 talents of gold. There were 12,000 garments of the Levites with their belts, and the *Ephod* – vest - and *Meil* – robe - of the *Cohen Gadol* – High Priest - which he wore when he performed the Temple service. In addition, there were 70,000 garments worn by the priests, with their belts, turbans and pants. David made all of these for them to atone for Israel. And the fittest men of Israel took them secretly, as they had been instructed. All of this service-gear was concealed until the future, to atone for Israel in the "End of Days."

Mishnah 9

"David also made 1,000 lyres and 7,000 harps to atone for Israel. He had cymbals for singing, extolling, thanksgiving, and praising the God of Israel, which was handed down to him from Moses, from Sinai...."

Color Plate 1-
Jacob's Dream

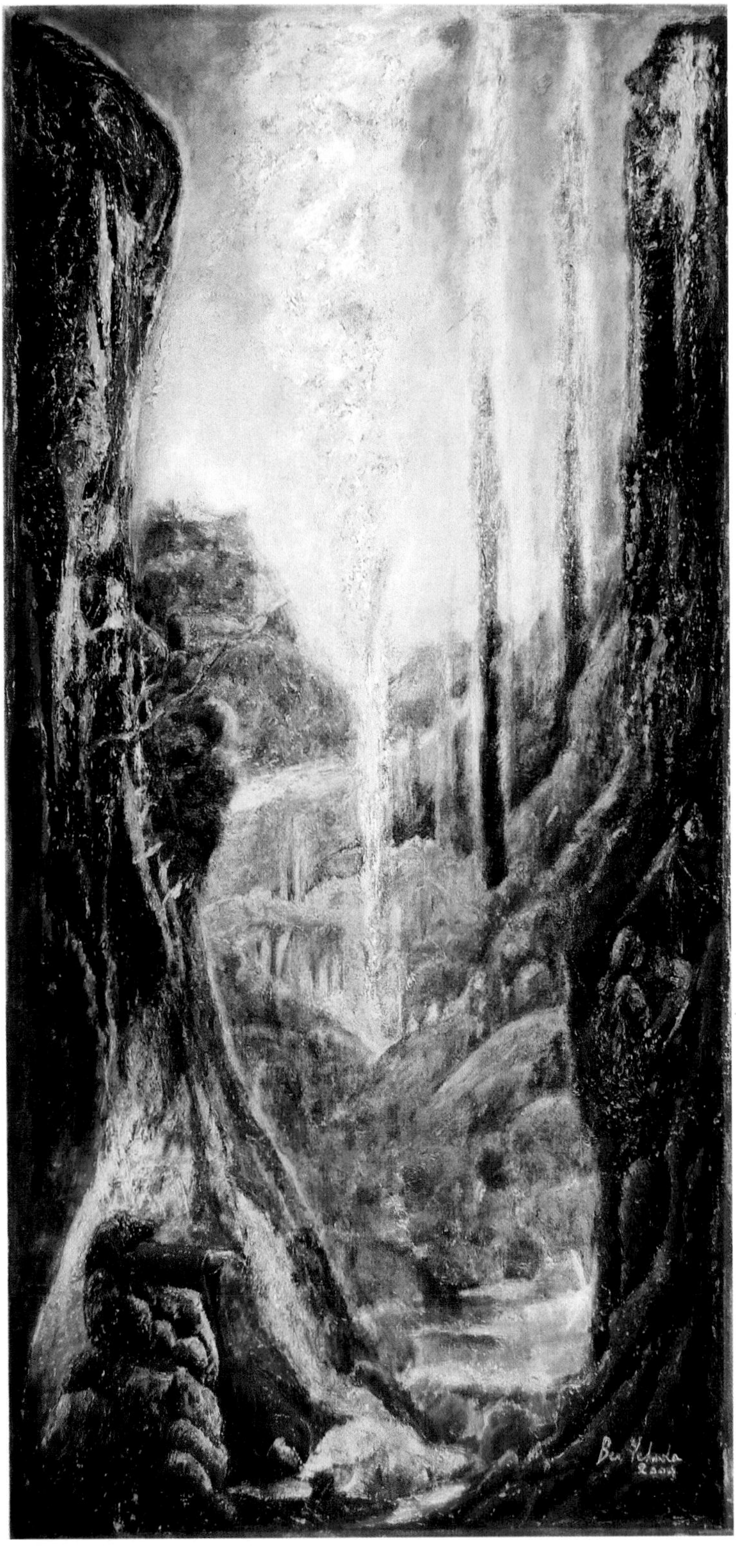

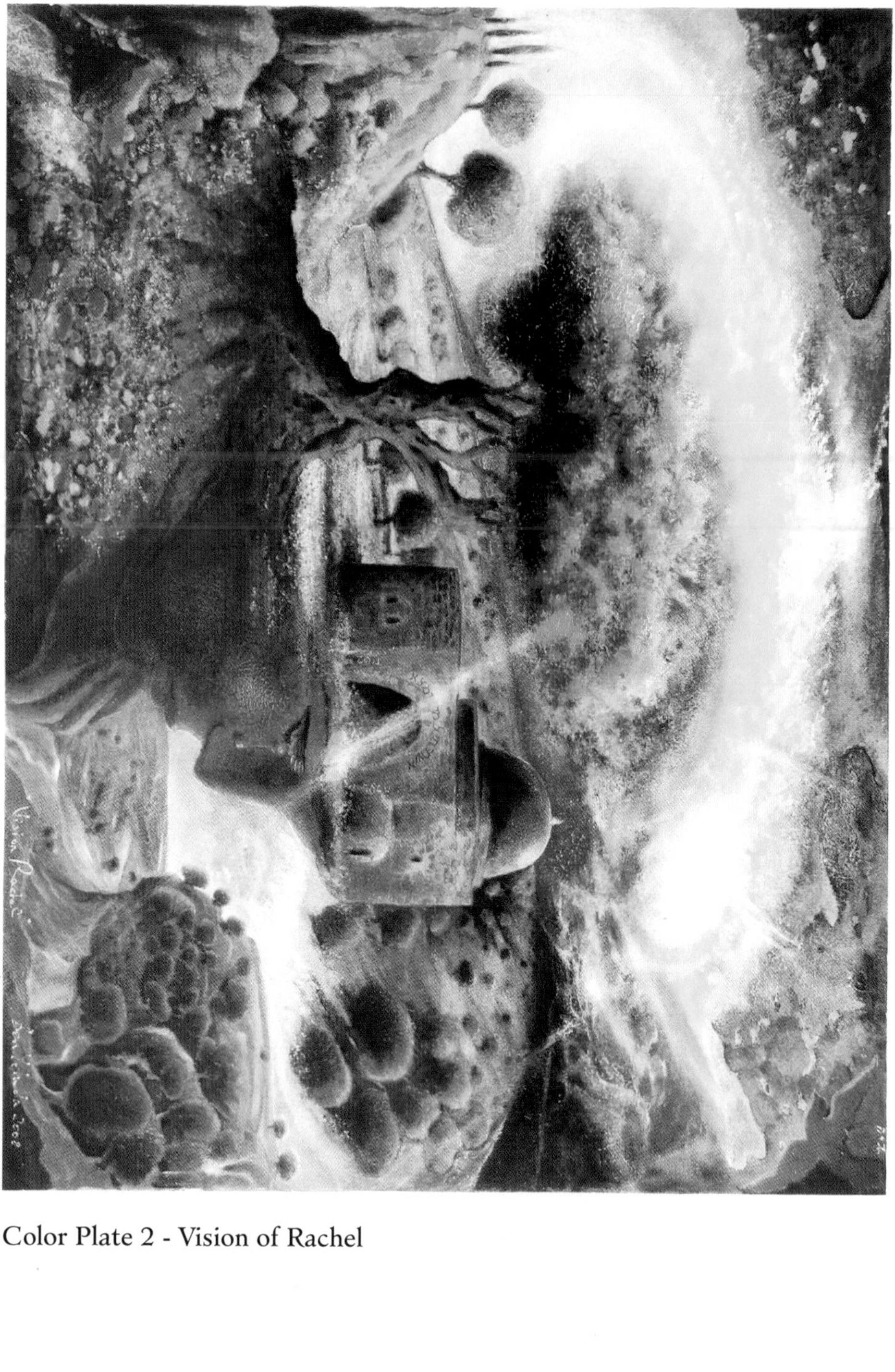

Color Plate 2 - Vision of Rachel

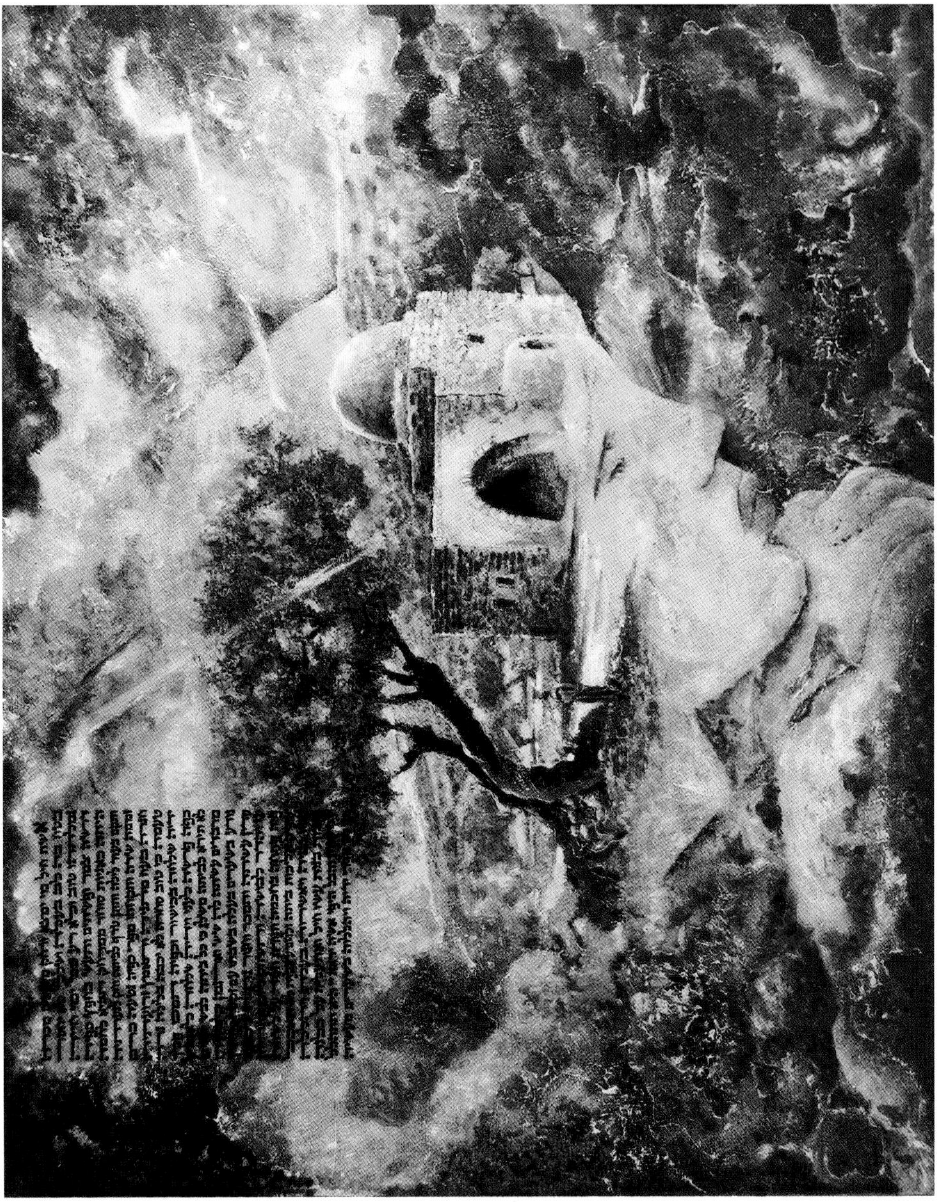

Color Plate 3 - Vision of Rachel #2

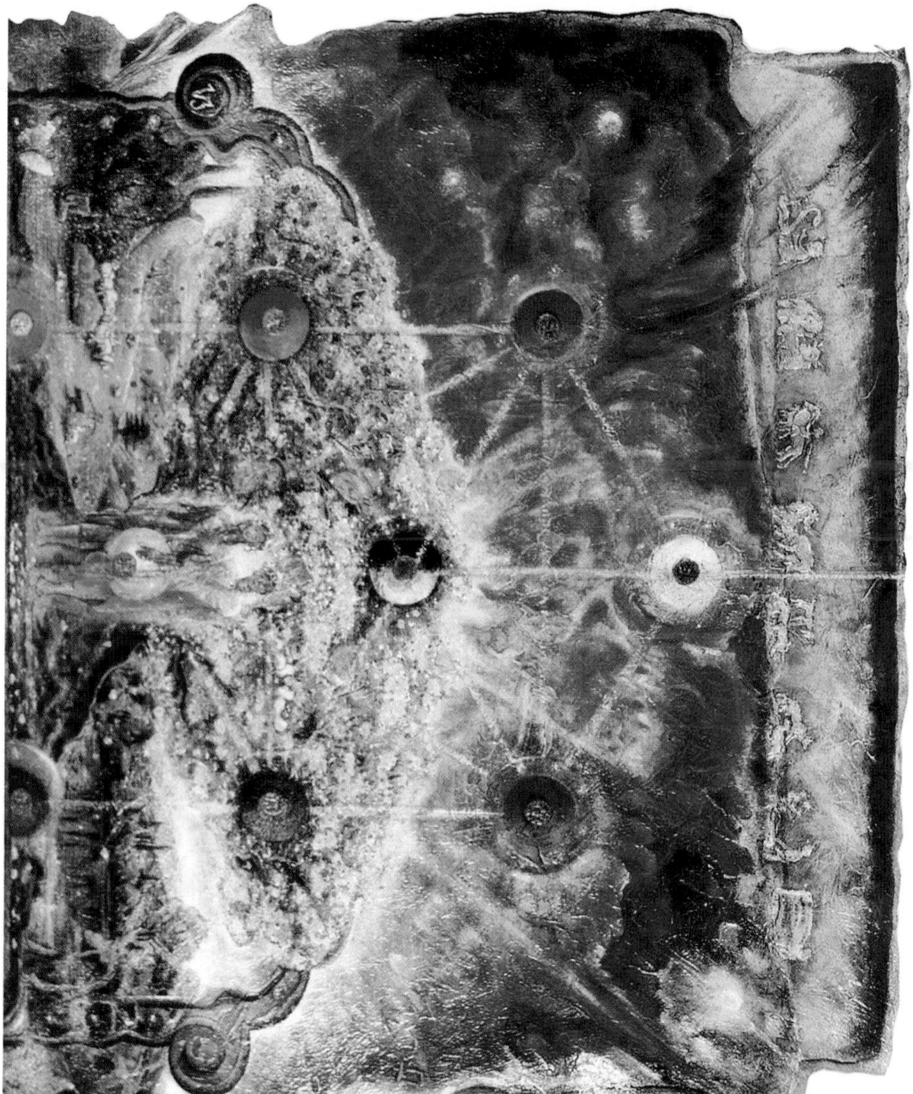

Color Plate 4 - The Tree of Life

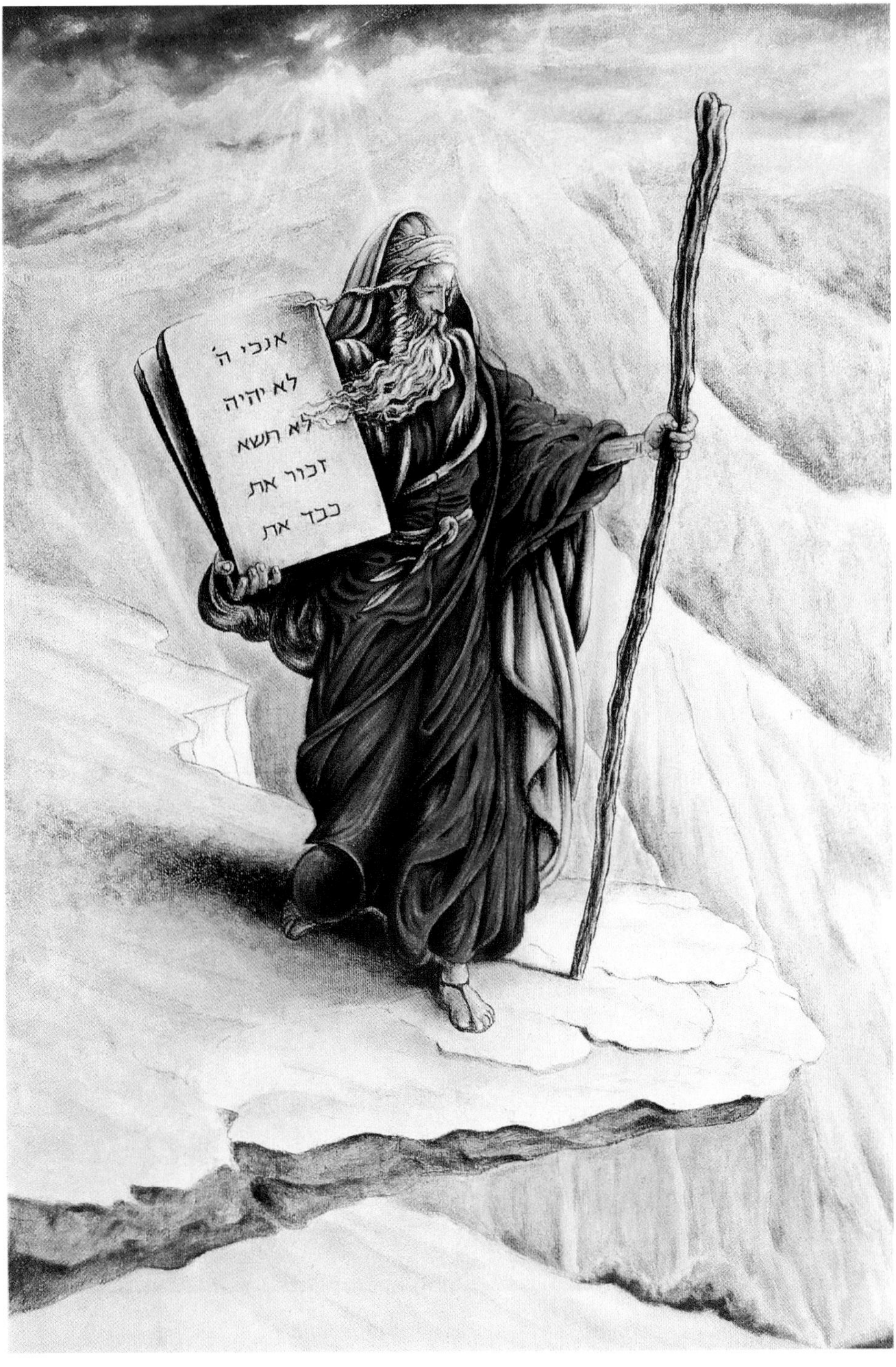

Color Plate 5 - Moses

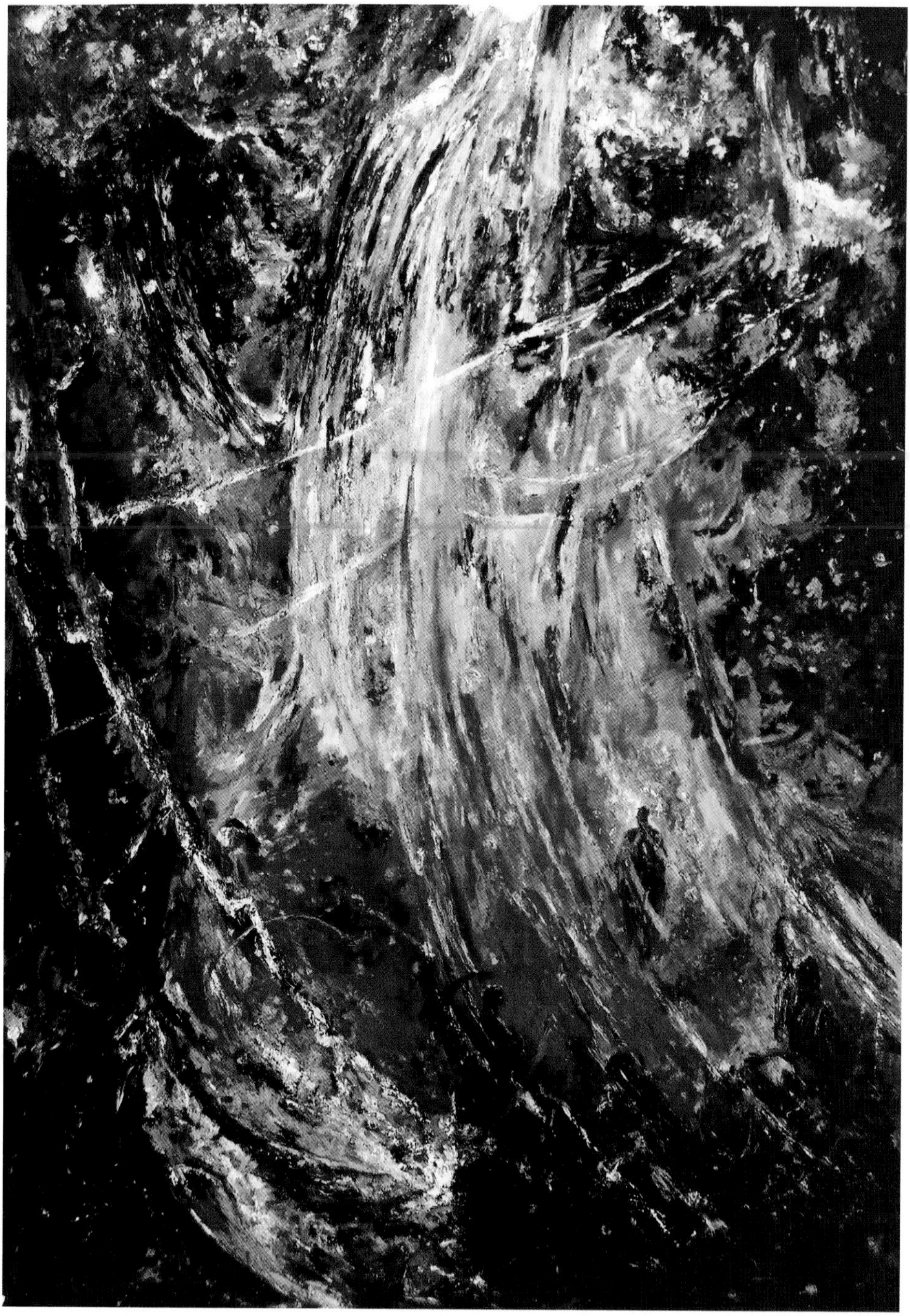

Color Plate 6 - The Great Day at Sinai

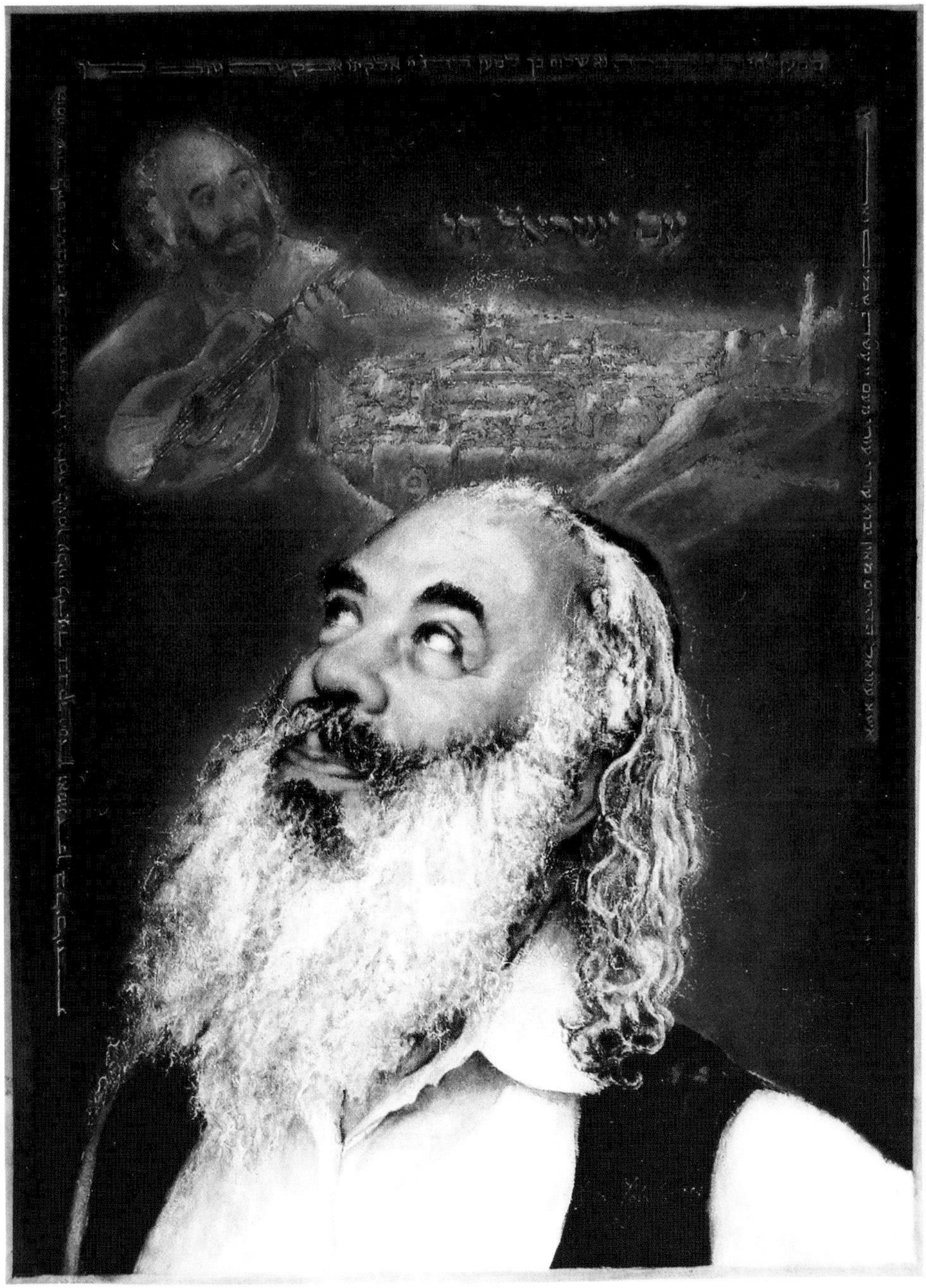

Color Plate 7 - 'Reb' Shlomo portrait

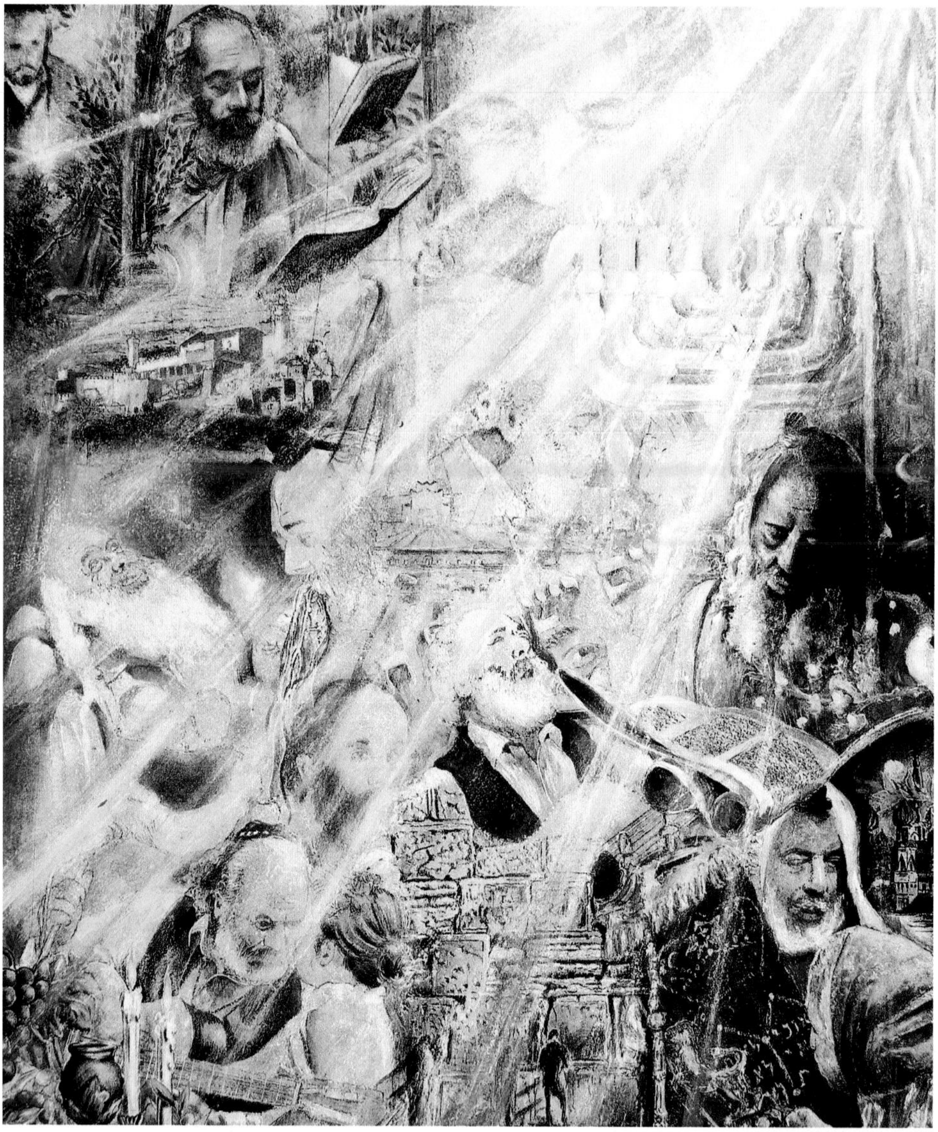

Color Plate 8 - 'Reb' Shlomo mosaic

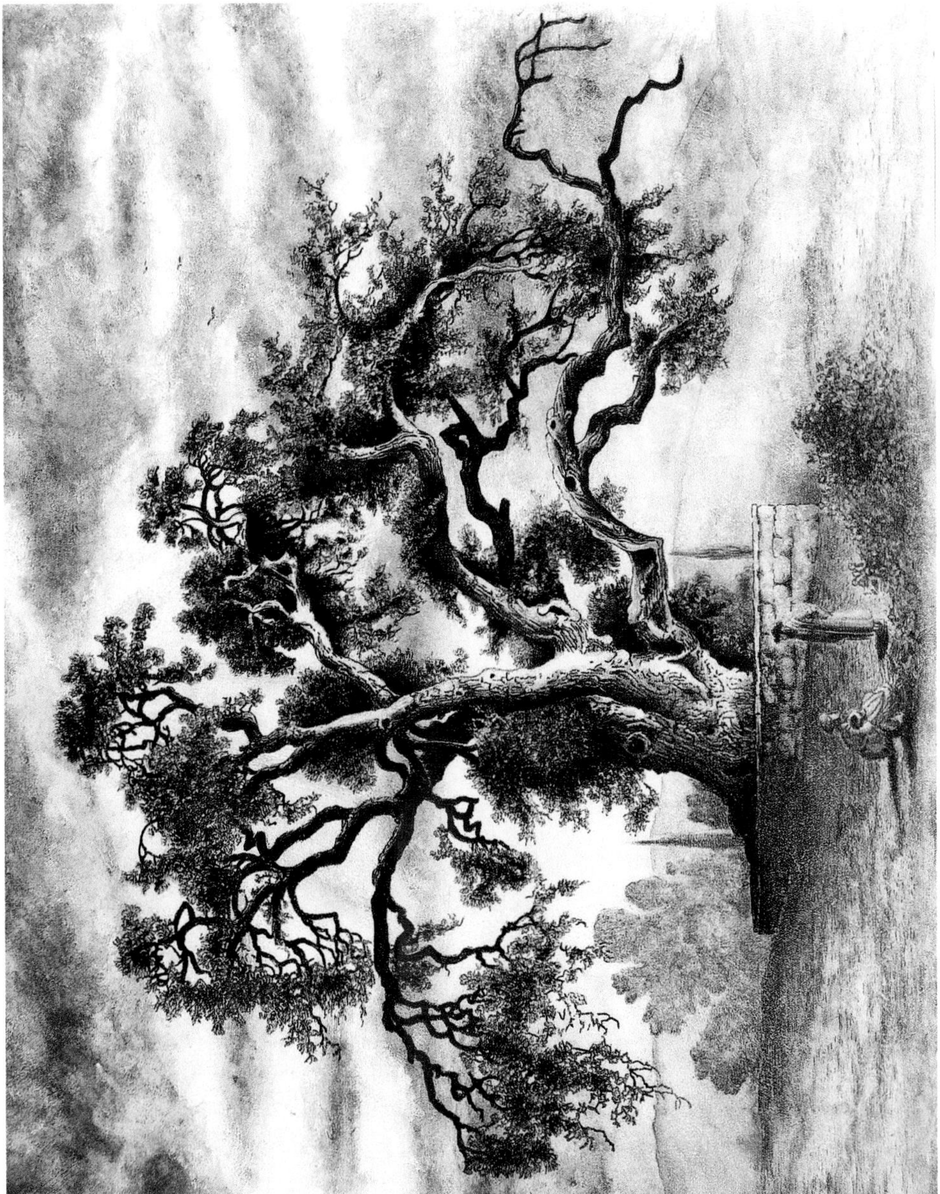

Color Plate 9 - The Oak of Abraham

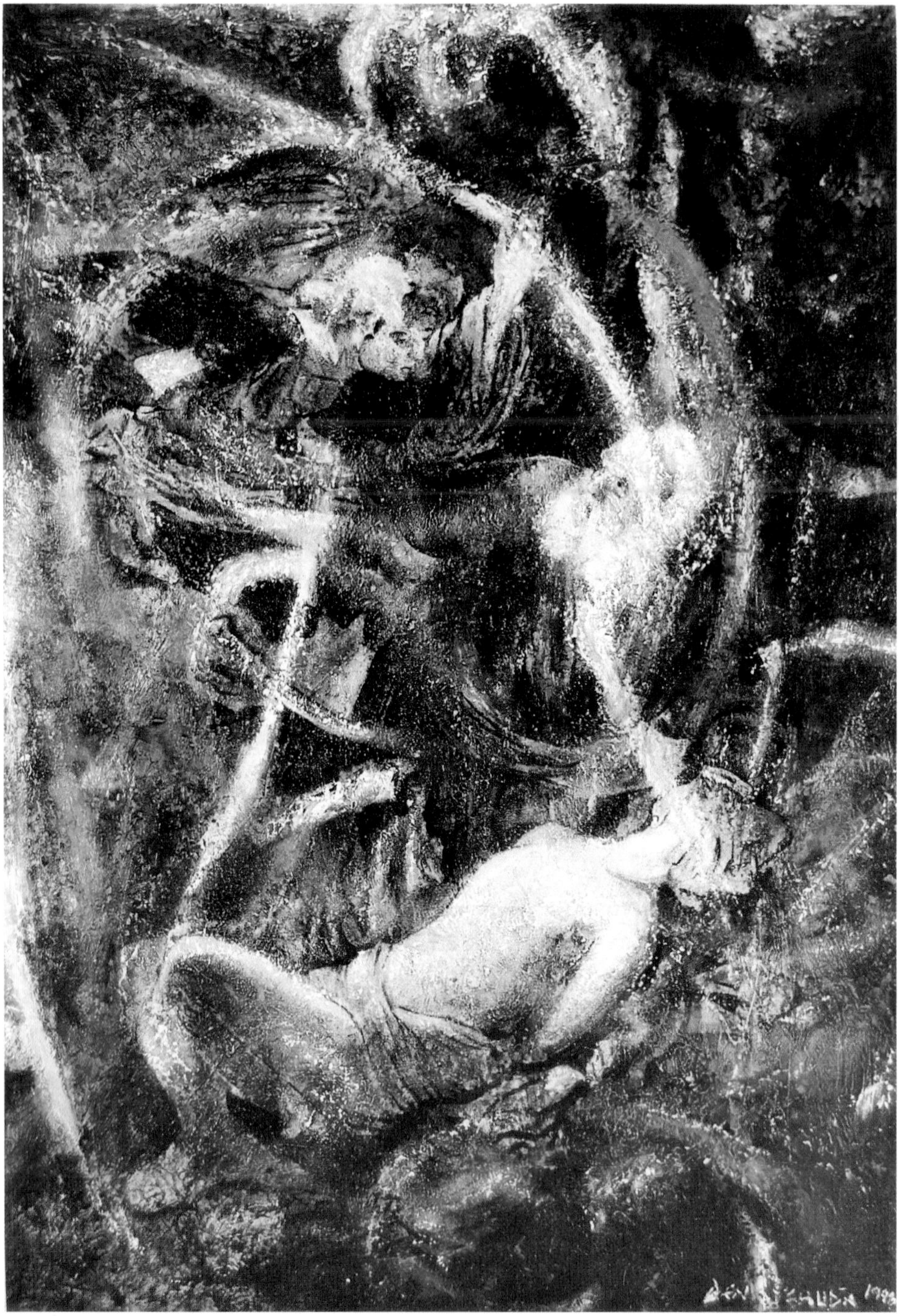

Color Plate 10 - The Sacrifice of Isaac

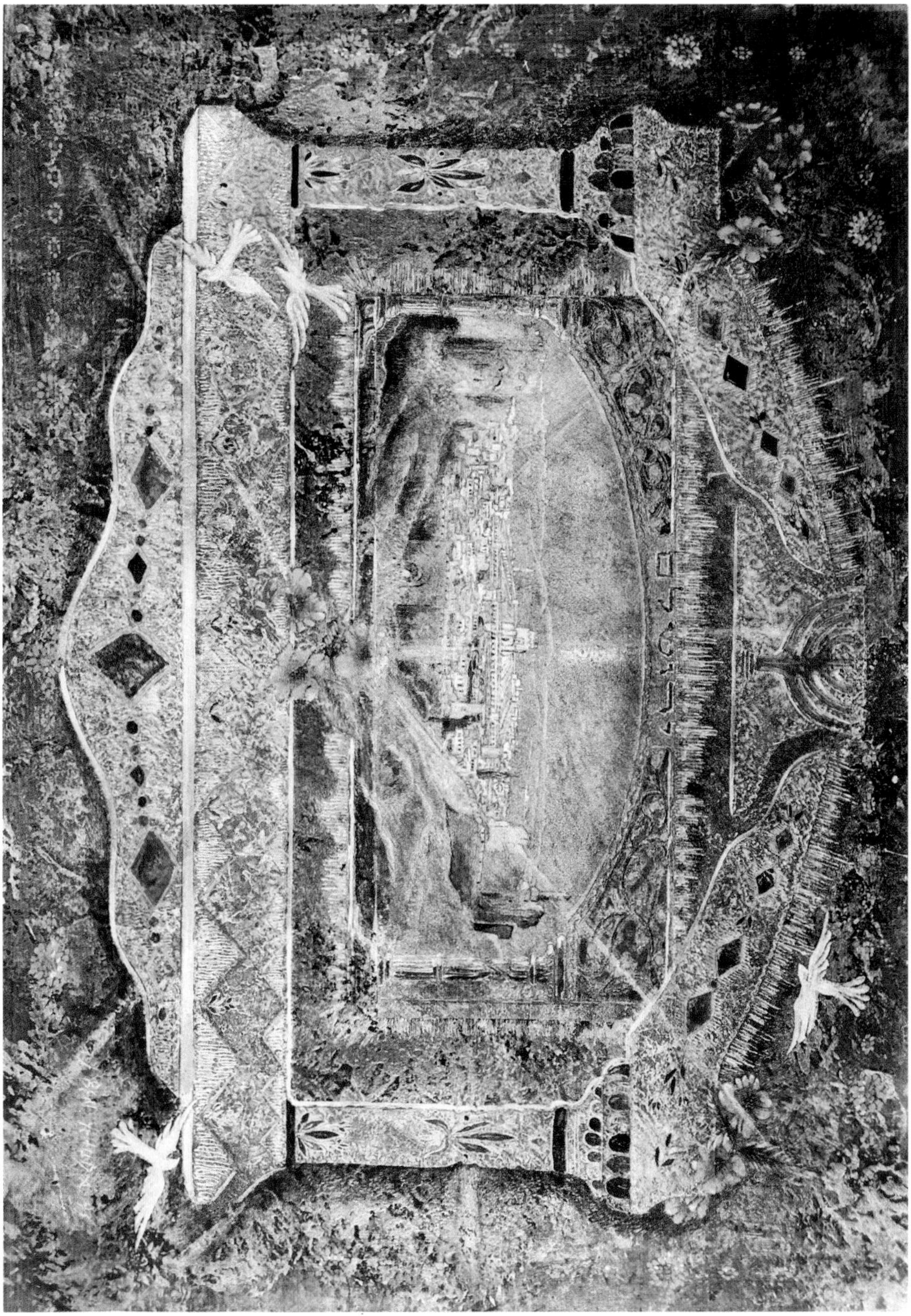

Color Plate 11 - Jerusalem

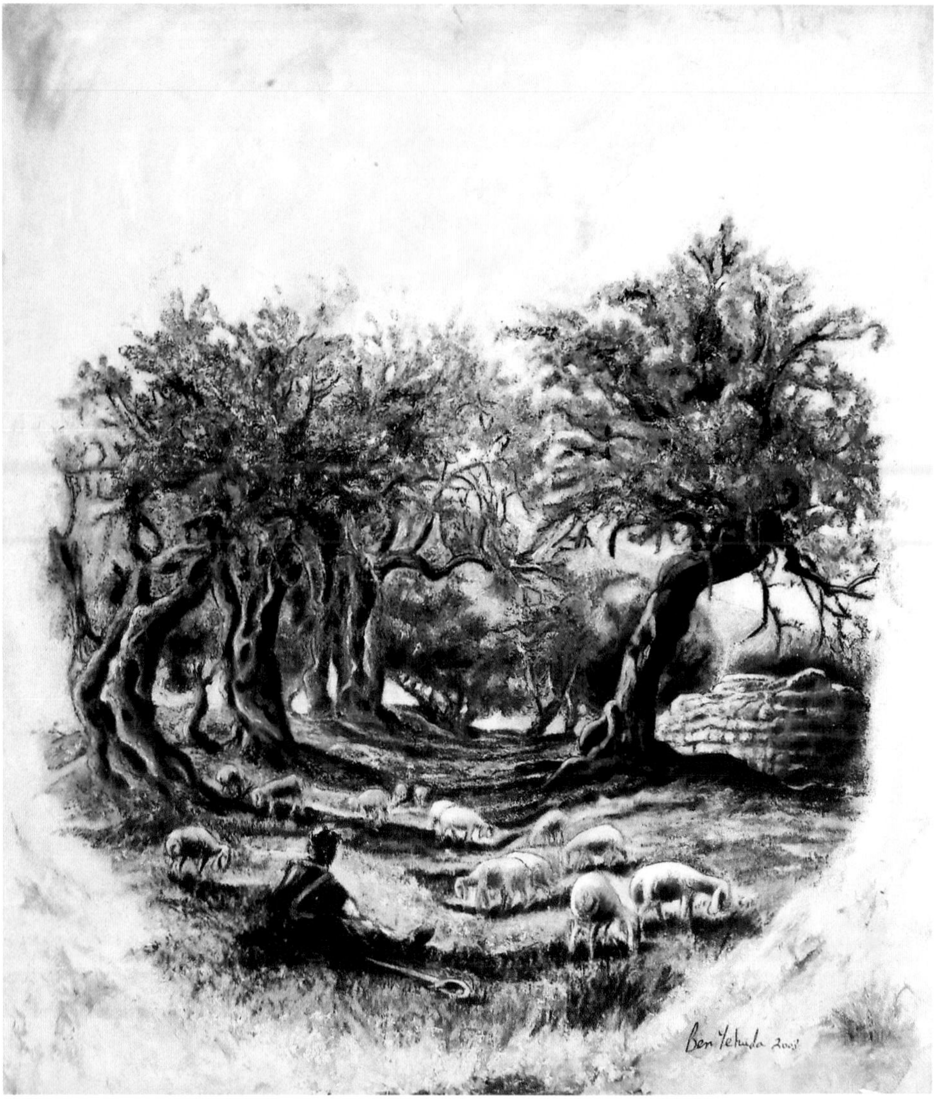

Color Plate 12 - The Youth David

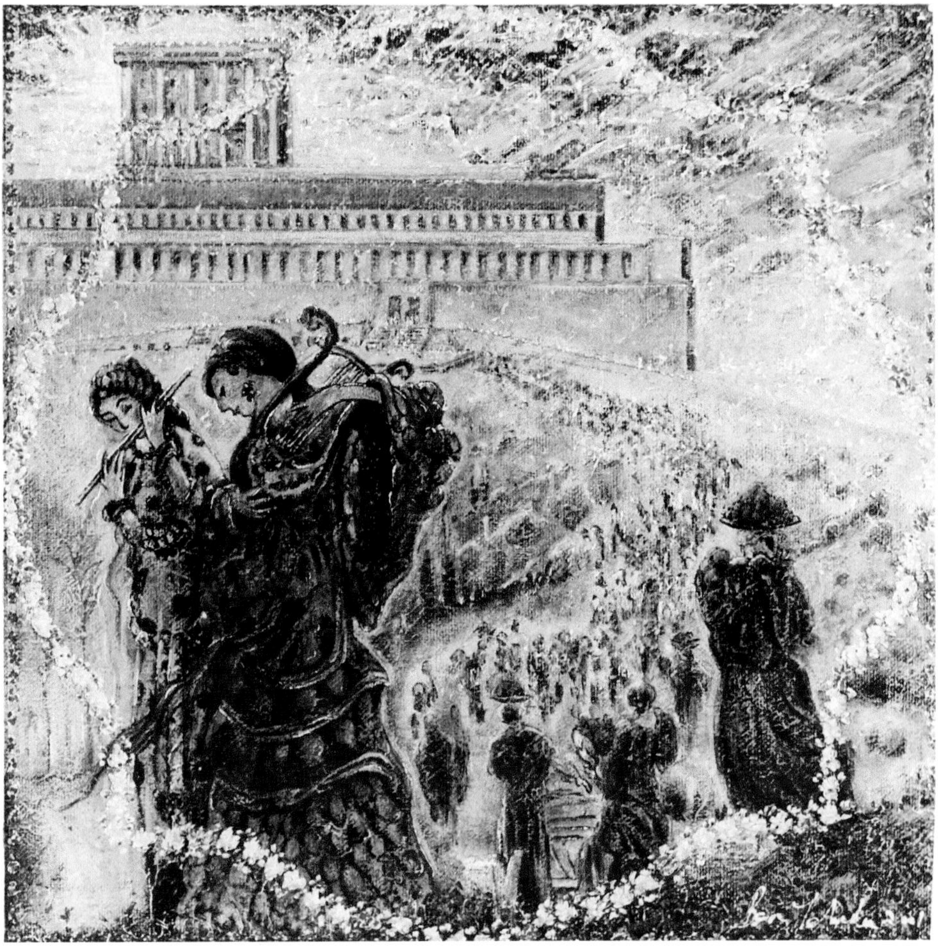

Color Plate 13 - Jerusalem Pilgrimage Festival

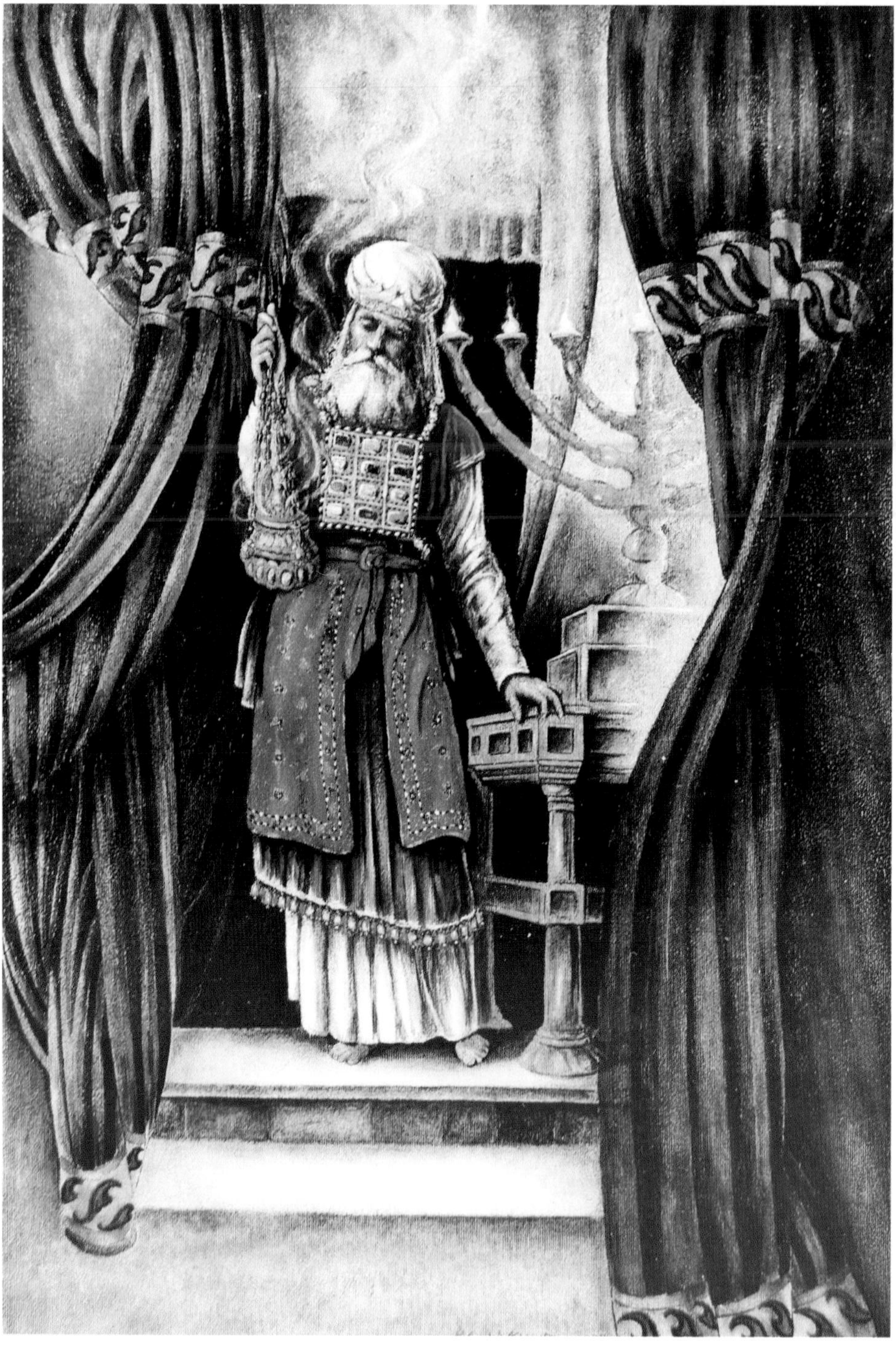

Color Plate 14 -The High Priest

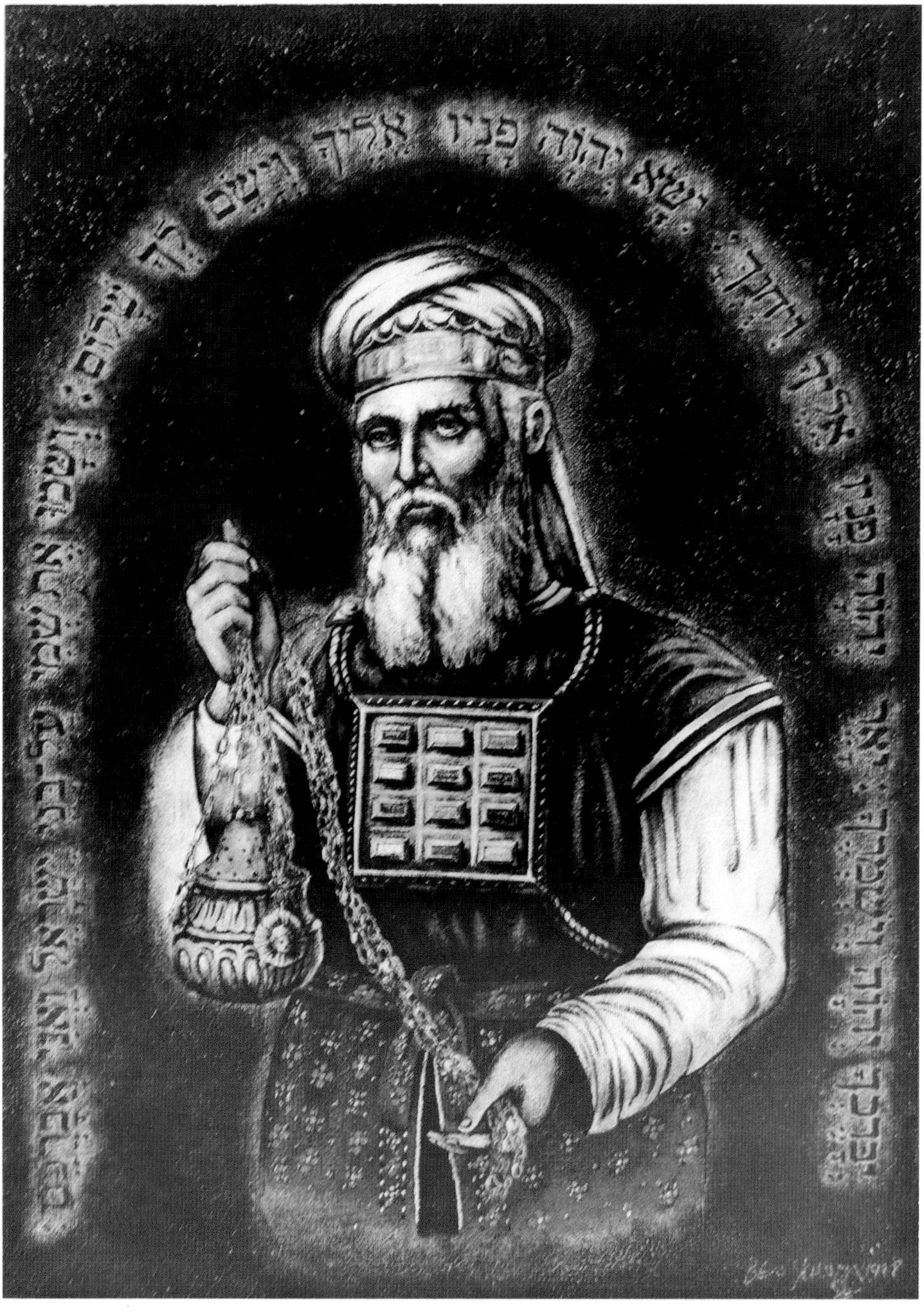

Color Plate 15 -The High Priest #2

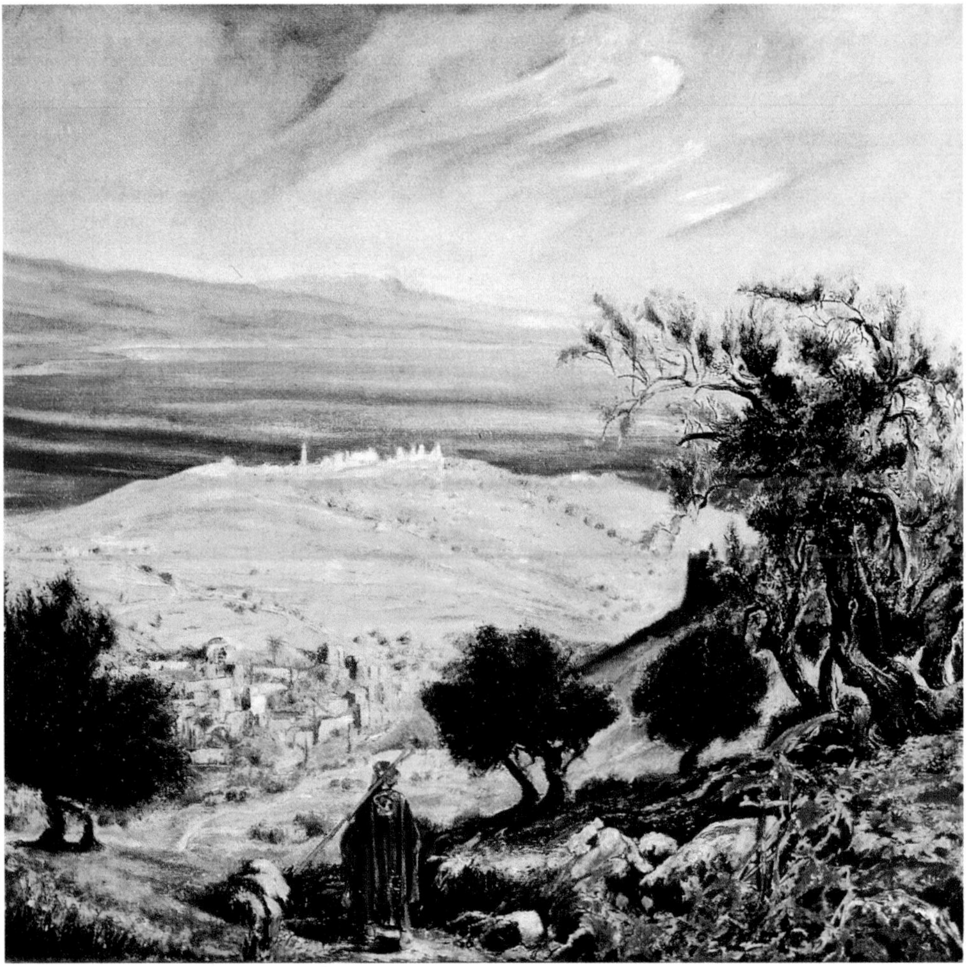

Color Plate 16 - The Sea of Galilee

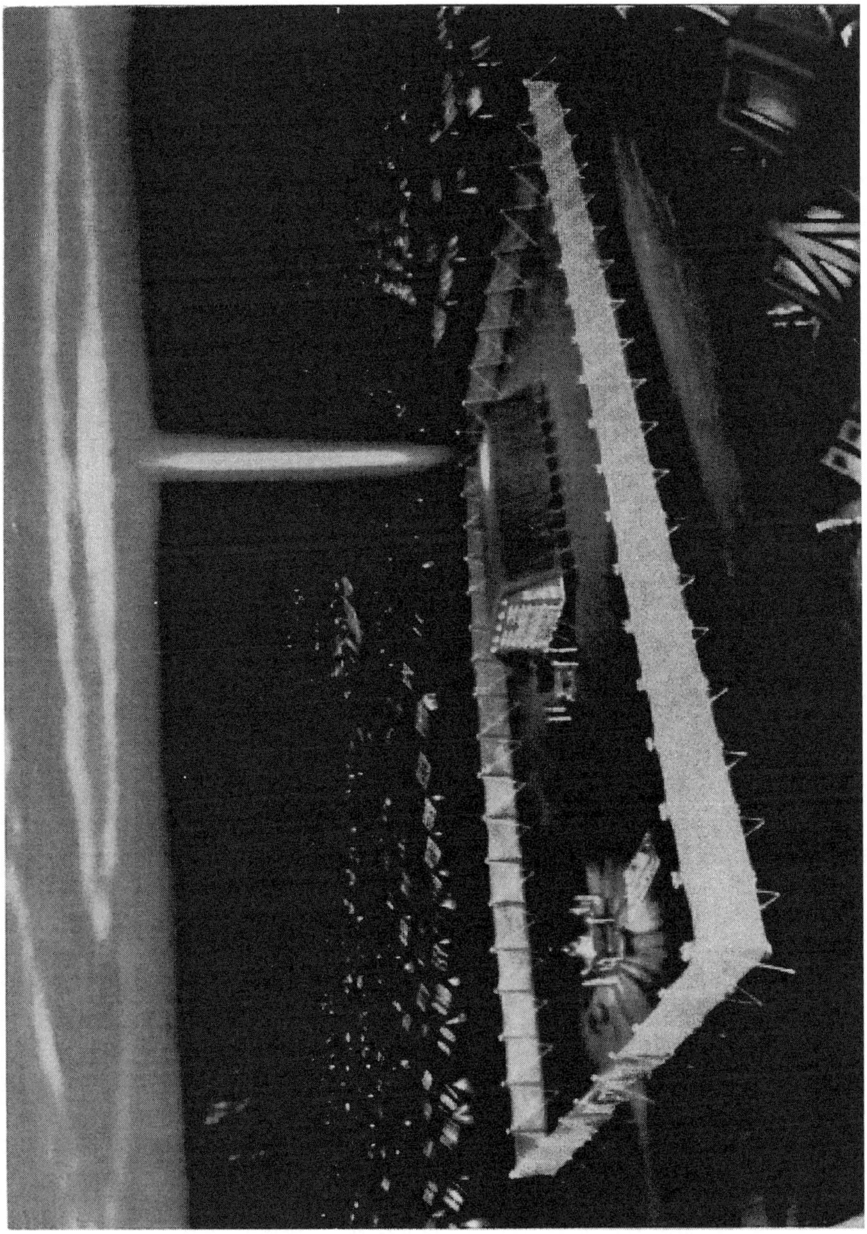

Plate 17 -The Desert Tabernacle

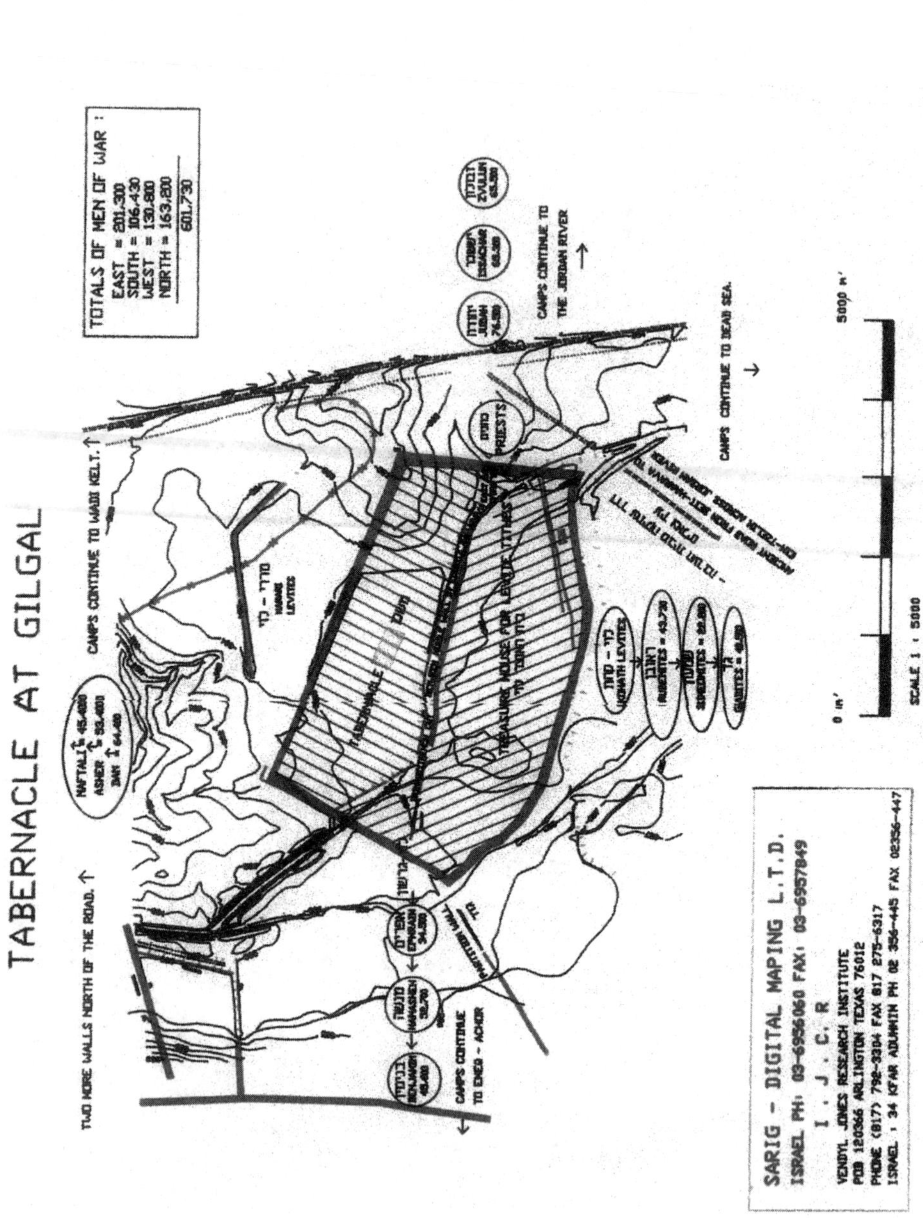

Plate 18 -The Tabernacle at Gilgal

Mystical Aromatherapy

Every person is divinely gifted with a unique body scent, a fragrant expression of our own body chemistry. Our personal scent becomes lovelier as we become more healthy and balanced. When we reach our ultimate goal of perfect health, our body scent will become extremely beautiful. Then we will all finally merge into One Heavenly Fragrance, identical to the Fragrance of the Garden of Eden and the Scent of the Temple Incense.

PART TWO

Hands-On Aromatherapy

Chapter 6

Sacred Aromatic Healing

Our ancient Judaic tradition reveals that according to the Divine Plan, certain botanicals created by the Holy One are potent medicines that bring the perfect healing we need, for virtually every type of ailment. The original aromatic plants of the Garden of Eden tend to have the most potent healing properties. True healing goes well beyond simply covering up or even eliminating the symptoms of ill health. Rather, it is a total rebalancing at the root of the ailment condition, an integration of all parts of a person's being, and ultimately a return to the original paradise state of elevated consciousness and radiant health.

Which fragrances bring the greatest healing? It all depends upon who is being treated. A total of about 750 aromatic constituents have been identified within the various botanicals of the plant kingdom. Many plants share common components, yet each is a different combination of these chemical building blocks, giving the plant a unique aroma and medicinal value. The potency, quality and therapeutic nature of each botanical is also somehow revealed in its particular fragrance.

There are many natural aromatic plants (and their highly concentrated essential oil extracts) to choose from, and the correct choices are most often quite different for each person. Also, the best choices for any individual will most often vary to some extent over time. The only exception to this might be the divinely ordained, enlightened remedy of the Temple incense. It is the "skeleton key of fragrance" that appears to be the best remedy for every person at any time. This master remedy perfectly incorporates all 11 "Sefirot" in the form of divinely revealed and heavenly prescribed holy spices, which represent the basic building blocks of all worlds. When properly combined together to make the incense, these elements are balanced and incorporated into one perfect medicine for all of humanity, and for all of life throughout time. It is the perfect fragrance of paradise.

The Temple incense, having power over death, appears to be the one fragrance that every soul remembers forever and is yearning for. It is the "missing link" that we all have in common: the quest of each soul to return to the Garden of Eden, the source of One-ness and life, the place of perfect fragrance. For this reason, the Temple incense is a model fragrance for study regarding the potential effects of aromatics on all of humanity. According to the late Rabbi Abraham Isaac Kook (HaCohen), who is recognized by many as the leading Judaic sage and mystic of our time, the Temple incense is the perfect link between the spiritual and physical worlds for every person.

We have a strong hint that aromatic botanicals have great healing potential, because the Temple incense has such vast healing powers. Any botanical that we are greatly attracted to aromatically shares a close relationship with the effect of the Ketoret, as it is also reminding us of, and bringing us back to, the Garden of Eden in our consciousness and physical health. Our fragrance preferences change because we change over time, particularly when we follow a proper diet and use herbal medicine effectively. Certain *klipot* - husks or outer shells - in our being fall away, like peeling away the outer layers of an onion. The actual goal is to get to the point where all of the husks have fallen away, to aid in the development of a healed, perfected being, a person said to be "on the level of the 11 spices of the incense."

Thus we can begin to comprehend the inner meaning of "oil and incense make the heart rejoice."[1] As we have learned, the "oil" refers to the guiding light of the Menorah, and "incense" to the Temple incense, which was ignited by the priest directly after lighting the Menorah. On the holistic healing level, the light of the "Menorah" is our higher consciousness, connected with the limbic brain, which helps to give healing guidance and direct the proper choice of "incense" as aromatic botanical medicine. Awakening the light of wisdom, we diagnose carefully, choose good herbal candidates, and access the limbic brain through the olfactory system to experience and select the appropriate medicine. We then must safely and effectively put the medicine to proper use to uplift, heal and return us to our place of perfection and paradise.

How Aromatherapy Works

What happens when we inhale the fragrance of an aromatic plant or essential oil? How do substances breathed in with the air affect us? To begin with, let's consider the various functions of the nose, explore the sense of smell, and investigate how the body actually responds to fragrance. This is a rather mysterious process, only vaguely understood by modern science.

The nose has 3 primary functions:

a. It filters, warms, and moistens the air breathed in, before it reaches the lungs.

b. It acts as a "sound box" to amplify the sounds made by the vocal cords.

c. It is the organ of olfaction (smell).

The nose is lined with mucous membrane which secretes half a liter of mucous a day, serving to moisten the air passing over it. During infection, or when the nose is irritated, as in cases of hay fever, the amount of mucous secreted increases, and we get a "runny nose." This membrane has a very rich blood supply, and warmth from the blood flowing through the large number of tiny capillaries raises the temperature of the air as it passes through the nose. Dust, pollen and bacteria are filtered out of the air by the thousands of miniscule hairs, known as *cilia* which line the membrane, reducing the risk of irritation to the lungs.

The nose is connected to a number of bony cavities called *sinuses*, and these act as resonators for the voice. Perhaps you have experienced the vibration in these cavities during a singing lesson, or when chanting "Aum" in a yoga class. When the nose is blocked, it affects the sound of the voice, because the resonance is interrupted. Infections present in the nose can be transmitted to the sinuses, giving rise to acute pain and headaches.

Smell is perceived by the olfactory cells which are embedded in the mucous membrane in the upper part of the nose. These cells are a specialized type of nerve cell or sensory neuron, specially adapted for this purpose. The cilia in this part of the nose are highly sensitive, and are actually an extension of the nerve fibers connecting with the olfactory cells. These cilia have their tips in the layer of mucous, and are able to detect the tiny chemical particles which give rise to the odor of any fragrances which enter the nose, but only after these fragrance particles have been dissolved in the mucous.

The receptors of our human sense of smell within our nasal cavity occupy an area of only 4 square cm, while certain animals have a much greater area (a dog has about 150 square cm of receptor area), thus giving most animals a much more refined and highly sensitive olfactory ability. The taste buds on our tongue are capable of experiencing only the aspects of sweet, salty, sour and bitter. All the rest is an olfactory experience. Thus a person who has a cold and "can't taste" food is often still able to experience these four taste sensations on the tongue, but unable to have the refined "gourmet" taste experience of a meal, or fully experience the delicate food fragrances, because they have no olfactory response.

Essential oils enter the nose in the form of gasses, as they evaporate when in contact with the air, and we inhale them in this evaporated form. The special cilia pass on to the olfactory cells whatever information they have picked up about the gasses passing through the nose. Each olfactory cell has a long nerve fiber called an *axon* leading out of the main body of the cell, which in turn picks up this information and passes it on to the brain. These "messages" are sent along the nerve fibers in the form of electro-chemical energy. In most of the nerves in the body, this passing of "messages" (or impulses) about our environment is done through the spinal cord, and from there to the brain. But in the case of these olfactory cells, the nerve fibers pass through a tiny bony plate at the top of the nose, and connect directly with the area of the brain known as the *olfactory bulb*, situated in the cerebral cortex. As a result, fragrance "messages" are passed on to the brain quickly and directly.

Because the cilia are in immediate contact with the source of the fragrance, and the olfactory cells connect directly with the brain, the sense of smell has a powerful and immediate effect on all the levels of a person's existence. This occurs because the area of the brain associated with smell is very closely connected with that part of the brain known as the *limbic area*, which is concerned with our emotions, memory, sexual drive, intuition, dreams etc. This is the part of the brain that is not so well understood by scientists today. The olfactory bulb also connects closely with the *hypothalamus*, and in turn the hypothalamus controls the *endocrine gland system* (the glands that govern growth, metabolism, reproduction and also such responses as fright, excitement, etc.).

Virtually every function of the body is controlled by the brain, by way of the central nervous system, the endocrine glands etc., and so any process that can send "messages" directly to the brain can be used to influence the physical body, our emotions, and even our higher consciousness. The implications of this far-reaching effect of the sense of smell, and our instant, powerful response to the fragrances that we experience, are extremely important keys which should carefully guide our practice of aromatherapy.

The sense of smell also imprints on our memory. Master aromatherapist Patricia Davis informs us that "the (limbic) area of the brain that registers smell is very closely connected to the area which is involved with memory, and both are situated in the 'oldest' part of our brain... the part that was already developed in our most primitive ancestors. This would seem to suggest an explanation of why perfumes and smells of all kinds can so powerfully and mysteriously trigger complete recall of past events and emotions."[2] These primitive brain development areas that Ms. Davis is referring to also parallel and reflect the Judaic teachings regarding man's experience in being cast out the Garden of Eden, but with a special gift that would recreate the fragrance, and fully reignite our ancient memory of paradise.

Master aromatherapist Valerie Ann Worwood reports that "during bodywork, when certain parts of the body are being manipulated, earlier events in this life, and in some cases 'past' lives, are often released and recalled... through hypnosis; through 'always knowing' as in the case of children; through 'suddenly realizing'; and through (various) bodywork (practices). There is *another route into the past, through aroma*, which can bring back memories, not only of earlier events in this life, but (also) in (past) lives experienced before."[3]

This teaching regarding past life experiences highlights an important point of Rabbi Burstein's message. He emphasized that by experiencing the 11 fragrances of the Temple incense spices, even smelling them individually, this would restore in us an ancient memory of the Temple days, which would "speed up" the rebuilding of the Temple. In the same way, as we experience the aromatic botanicals that assist in our health care, we are reminded of our first experience with them in Paradise. Even after our long exile, everyone is still fully capable today of speeding up their return to an ancient past life in the Garden of Eden, through aroma.

Chapter 7

Essential Oils: Potent Botanical Medicine

Essential oils are extracted from aromatic plants, and they are by far the most highly concentrated and potent form of herbal medicine. Their proper use can often be the most effective approach to natural healing. Fragrant plants are covered with tiny sacks, containing volatile (evaporative) essential oil infused with life force. Present as tiny droplets captured in specialized cells which evolved to contain them, these aromatic molecules are saved in the plant for emergency use, as energy reserves and as an attractant for potential pollinators. They protect the plant against change of climate, disease and other environmental challenges. Similarly, these same fragrant oils tend to work within the human body in a balancing and protective manner, assisting our delicate life-support systems. The oils occur in aromatic herbs, grasses, leaves, rhizomes, flowers, citrus peels, core woods, resins, barks and roots.

Each aromatic botanical upon extraction yields a super-concentrated oil (on average, 30 grams of plant material yields only 1 drop), with a unique chemistry and distinct fragrance "personality" or soul. This is a vivid expression of the spirit of the plant - incorporating both medicinal and aromatic characteristics. When the soul fragrances speak to our own soul, and we receive pleasure from the experience, there is a soul-to-soul connection made which brings healing, balance and radiant life. Our holy tradition indicates that when this connection and union is made, *we also heal the plant*, since the plant kingdom was involved and somehow complicit in the "original sin." This is because the plant is now being used for the noble purpose of healing and returning us to the Garden, instead of driving us out.

Any substance that is inhaled in the air will be involved in a process of "gas exchange" in the lungs, and this particularly applies to all varieties of essential oils. Differing amounts of various oils dissolve in the bloodstream, depending on the nature, volatility and chemical structure of that particular oil. Part of the inhaled aromatic substance may be exhaled right away with the next breath, while the rest passes into the bloodstream. Blood circulates around the body at surprising speed – it takes only about 30 seconds to complete one circuit. As a result, substances dissolved into the lungs, or any other part of the bloodstream throughout the body, are absorbed in the particular relevant organs that they are drawn to, and can take effect very quickly.

Essential oils which are inhaled are thus almost instantly delivered by the bloodstream to various parts of the body. In any aromatherapy treatment which involves massage, bath or inhalation, some of the oil will be inhaled and taken in with the breath, and thus become effective almost immediately. With a massage or bath treatment, some oil will also be taken in via absorption through the skin. This has the advantage of simultaneously delivering both a quick-acting and a slow-acting effect. However, when oils are taken by mouth, they don't have the direct brain connection, and can take longer to act as they slowly reach the bloodstream, transported through the digestive system. Taking oils orally by any person – or under the guidance of any person – who is untrained or improperly trained can be a very dangerous practice, as most essential oils can severely burn the mouth or throat.

While some essential oils exercise a general healing effect on the whole organism, others exhibit a special affinity for a particular organ or body system. These will have a specific effect on that organ or system when the oil or blend reaches that region, and by nature concentrates there, in its circulating journey. The correctly chosen essential oils will amazingly go right to work in the targeted destination. Usually the oils work effectively in the body for about three days, after which time they are naturally eliminated.

After the body has received the therapeutic benefits, any remaining residue of essential oil may be excreted through the skin as sweat, or may be returned to the lungs to be exhaled with the breath. Oils which have an affinity with the kidneys will be excreted primarily in the urine, while oils which have an affinity for the lungs will mainly be exhaled with the breath. Being knowledgeable about these affinities enables the therapist to select the most effective essential oil(s) for a specific treatment. For example, there are many oils with antiseptic properties. However, knowing that oil of rose has a special affinity with the uterus and the female reproductive system, that frankincense oil has an affinity with the lungs, or that chamomile and bergamot oils relate in particular to the urinary tract, guides the therapist. This aids in selecting the oil(s) that are most effective in the treatment of various organs or ailments, such as cystitis, bronchitis or a uterine infection. Other oils are much more wide-ranging and many of them often have a more general healing effect on the entire body.

The processes by which plants "manufacture" essences are very similar to those by which they produce food for the plant's growth, and other substances necessary for the life and health of the plant. Naturally occurring chemical elements in the soil, water and air are broken down and put together by the plant in many different combinations. The energy needed to fuel these chemical changes comes from the sun, and the plant's manufacturing process is known as photosynthesis. Aromatic plants produce essential oils in special cells, usually near the surface. The oil may be stored within the secretor gland, or the plant may develop some special structure such as a pocket or duct in which the oil is collected near the secretor cells. The way in which the oil is stored in the plant makes it easier or more difficult to extract it, and determines the best extraction method and procedure.

Essential Oil Extraction Methods

The type of plant material and its composition often determine which type of extraction is chosen to produce the best quality essential oil, Absolute or CO_2 extract.

1. **Distillation** is the most basic and common extraction technique used today. The practice of distillation originates from ancient alchemical principles, and it was considered to be one of the magical arts. This "secret" process was discovered and lost several times throughout history in several advanced cultures. Our modern form traces its history from the Arabic physician, alchemist and philosopher Avicenna (980–1037). Since his rediscovery, the equipment that has been used has taken several forms, although the distillation always takes place in 3 stages: separation, purification and recombination. The forms are:

   a. *Water Distillation*. The plant material is placed in a kettle, covered with water and boiled. Steam vapors are condensed and collected; the essential oil rises to the top and is decanted off.

   b. *Water and Steam Distillation*. Similar to above, except that the plant material is suspended on a grille above the boiling water, and steam from a boiler is forced through the kettle.

c. *Steam Distillation*. This is the most common form today. The plant material is put in a kettle without water, and steam from a boiler is forced through.

In distillation, two different aromatic products are obtained: The distillate water, known as a *hydrosol*; and the *essential oil* that floats to the top of this water. The hydrosol has a short shelf life and should be refrigerated. It contains the aromatic parts of the plant material that are water soluble, and is valuable cosmetically, in health care as an aromatic room spray, and occasionally in culinary use.

2. **Cold Pressure Extraction** is used to extract citrus oils from the fruit skins of lemon, lime, orange, grapefruit, tangerine, mandarin, and bergamot. Basically the skins are put into a huge hydraulic press. After squeezing at high pressure, the citrus essential oil is decanted off the top of the extract, and carefully filtered to remove any sediment.

3. **Solvent Extraction** is a two-step process using volatile chemical solvents such as hexane or benzene. It has been employed for the past 50 years or so to obtain the precious extracts of delicate flowers and other aromatic materials, some of which cannot withstand the heat of the distillation process. A complete extract with a fragrance similar to the original aromatic material is produced. In the first step, essential oil and plant waxes are extracted together from the aromatic material, to form a waxy semi-solid product known as the *Concrete*. Then special equipment is used with an alcohol wash to remove the waxes, and extract the final aromatic product, known as an *Absolute*. If the process is done correctly, virtually all of the volatile solvent and waxes are removed.

4. **CO_2 Extraction** is a newly developed process that produces perhaps the very best quality oils. The product is a total extract similar to an Absolute, but without the use of any chemical solvents. When carbon dioxide is pressurized without heat in very specialized equipment, it acts like a liquid and extracts the aromatic oil, which is obtained when the pressure is released. Another big advantage is that any chemicals or impurities in the plant material are suppressed, producing a remarkably clean, highly aromatic material, a "CO_2 extract."

Essential Oil Quality: Naturals vs. Synthetics

Many different qualities of aromatic oils are sold in the marketplace. Some are natural essential oils, but most are synthetic fragrances which are not of natural origin. In fact, most fragrances sold today are synthetic lab-made chemicals, and are quite poisonous. These toxic materials can not be naturally processed by the body, so collect in the liver, along with other poisons from our intake of food, air and water. When our toxicity level gets too high we become ill, sometimes with a very serious ailment. To protect our health, it is best to completely avoid any products containing these dangerous synthetic fragrances, and any other toxins, from whatever source.

Over the past 75 years, the pursuit of costly, rare and often unavailable true botanical essential oils has led to a rapidly expanding and highly profitable industry in these poisonous "aroma-chemicals." By clever manipulation of molecular structure, these petroleum refinery products are re-constructed in the lab by fragrance chemists to create an enormous array of trendy product scents. Recent advances in this field of aroma-chemistry have flooded the market with mass-produced low-cost imitation fragrances, which are the basis of most of the perfumes and cosmetics sold today (ranging from the most expensive to the cheapest varieties), and countless other food and non-food household products.

Why are these synthetic chemicals mass-produced and so widely sold? The main reason is financial. They are extremely profitable, as they are so very cheap to produce. For example, to mass-produce imitation "rose oil," the cost is about $3.00 per kg, but to produce natural rose oil (steam distilled "rose otto"), the cost can range as high as $10,000.00 per kg - three thousand times the price of the synthetic imitation!

Your ability to distinguish between the naturals and synthetics is the first step in determining the medicinal value (if any) of an aromatic product. The best way to know if you are smelling a medicine or a poison, aside from reliable but very expensive lab testing, is to develop your nose to recognize natural oils, and the presence of synthetics. This may take years of experience. There are also other important criteria you can reliably follow. Natural oils are sold only in dark or colored bottles, they have a widely varying range of prices, and important information should be presented including the Latin botanical name, the part(s) of the plant used, and the country of origin. Be careful about any aromatic oil or blend that is being presented with a romantic theme, as this is a common ploy used by the synthetics industry to seduce and confuse a consumer. Otherwise, you would really need to know your producer, carefully study the production process and the ingredients used – and preferably get the product directly from the producer or his direct reliable agent whenever possible.

To be on the safe side, assume that most aromatic commercial products are (or contain) synthetic chemical fragrance(s), unless you know otherwise. Occasionally you will find products scented with true natural citrus, as these oils are relatively inexpensive to produce. In this case the product will often proudly state that it contains "natural fragrance." You still need to be careful, because it might also contain a certain per cent of aroma-chemicals.

In spite of the immediate and far-reaching nature of our olfactory response, our usual daily awareness of the sense of smell is generally less consistent than our other senses. It is so much more subtle. Also, our perception of smell decreases very quickly if the same aroma is inhaled for more than a very short period, and in fact the fragrance may very soon become completely undetectable. This strange phenomenon is known as *fading*. You are witnessing it when you walk into the kitchen and remark, "What smells so good?" - only to find that the cook, who has been in the kitchen all along, cannot smell anything special at all! For your nose, the apple pie is a wonderful new fragrance, and therefore powerfully experienced, but for the baker, "fading" has already taken place. The very same effect easily occurs whenever any types of aromatics are experienced.

So, when we come in contact with natural essential oils, the fragrance can fade out very quickly. This phenomenon is evident whenever the oils are in the air; when we have applied them to the skin as a perfume; during a massage or bath treatment; and also when we smell the oils on a tissue, fragrance strip or directly from the bottle. This is the primary reason why we try to keep the choice of sampled fragrances down to just a few oils – the nose fades out. Synthetic, "man-made" aromatic chemicals are much more intense, and are lab designed to have far greater tenacity and *not* fade out. Oddly, people who are involved with the use of synthetic fragrances will often feel that a natural essential oil application is fragrantly very weak and "poor quality," partly because all too soon the natural scent just fades away.

Natural vs. Synthetic Medicine

This is a key area in which natural medicines such as true essential oils differ from the synthetic pharmaceutical "medicines" of the large drug manufacturers. In recent years, pharmaceutical companies have shown renewed interest in what they call "botanicals" (drugs of plant origin), but they have failed to understand the holistic principles underlying the successful use of whole plant medicines. Having identified a single active component from a plant, they isolate this component and use it alone to treat a specific symptom. Sometimes this component is taken from a plant, but usually it is synthesized in a factory. Chemists try to put together molecules which match those of the original plant material, using the same range of elements that the plant uses.

But it is the very complex nature of plant remedies, with their many active components - each one balancing and supplementing the other – that makes a plant medicine unique, and accounts for the rarity of unwanted side-effects. The many elements in an essential oil act in symbiosis with each other. Ironically, what the drug manufacturers see as "impurities" are the very components that are vitally needed in combination with the drug component they have extracted or copied, to ensure its safe and successful use.

Range of Quality Among Natural Essential Oils

After the synthetic chemical fragrances are eliminated from consideration as safe medicines or aromatics, the next step is to determine the quality of the natural essential oils available. Almost all natural essential oils are mass-produced and designed to be used in the food and flavor industry. These oils are not of a high enough quality standard for aromatherapy use, as they are very limited therapeutically and aromatically, and often contain large amounts of agricultural chemicals. Some of these inexpensive oils wind up on the shelves of many stores. You will save money on them, but as with most products, you will only get what you pay for - in this case, a product that might be used to fragrance herbal potpourris, at best.

In addition, some "natural" fragrances are actually custom designed in the lab, reconstructed partly or entirely from components of other natural oils. This is done for financial reasons, to cut down on production costs and expand inventory. For example, it is well-known in the industry that France annually exports three times the amount of Lavender oil than is distilled. These "man-manipulated" compounded oils have no place in professional aromatherapy practice, and should be avoided. Be determined to obtain the very highest quality essential oils available, if they are to be used therapeutically.

What Conditions Produce a Quality Essential Oil?

These are the vital elements: proper soil and fertile cultivation fit for the species; healthy seeds; proper germination and plant maintenance; ideal climate conditions for the type of plant, including the optimal amount of water and sunlight; proper harvesting practices including correct harvest timing, and - for most species - correct drying technique, and in particular drying time; careful distillation with the right type of equipment. In particular, the distiller must be careful not to "burn" the plant material through excessive "overcooking." And finally, the resulting essential oil must be kept sterile, not adulterated in any way, properly bottled and correctly stored.

How can we gather reliable information about the quality? It is possible to scientifically test oils with specialized equipment, a process known as GLC (gas liquid chromatography). These tests are quite expensive; however they accurately and reliably compare the components of a sample to a known standard for that oil. The cost is worthwhile in certain cases, especially when the sample tested is taken from a much larger quantity of essential oil.

The best way to immediately recognize a high quality essential oil is by carefully developing and educating your sense of smell. Train yourself by gently responding to and comparing essential oils from different sources which are assumed to be of high quality. A sensitive and trained nose will detect an entire symphony of fragrance in every quality oil, experiencing each natural component as a note of fragrance in a wave of perfect harmony.

Professionally speaking, it takes about 20 years for most people to develop the sensitivity, and become fluent in the olfactory language, to fully experience a fragrance and describe it eloquently. Achieving that, one's peers respectfully endow a fragrance master with the distinction of being called a "Nose!"

Organic vs. Non-Organic Essential Oils

The very highest quality essential oils are produced from plants grown organically, or wild harvested, under optimal conditions in every respect. It is important that the plants have had no exposure to agricultural chemicals or other poisons from any source. In organic agriculture as it applies to essential oils, only organic fertilizers are used, with no chemical fertilizers added to the soil. There is a total restriction on the use of all chemical pesticide sprays. In addition, the plants must grow in a pollution-free area, protected from any exposure to toxins nearby. An Organic certifying agency usually requires that a chemical-free environment must be maintained for a minimum of five years before the plants can be documented as being truly organic.

It is very important that the plants have absolutely no contact at all with any chemical toxins, such as agricultural fertilizers or sprays, because these poisons invariably wind up in the essential oils in large concentrations upon extraction. The toxins are released from the plant material during the steam distillation process, together with tiny droplets of essential oil. Since the chemicals are mostly *not water-soluble*, they rise to the top of the distillate hydrosol water and become mixed together with the essential oil floating on top. The toxic chemical concentration in non-organic essential oils thus **much** greater than the concentration in the original plant material, because the oils are such a concentrated extract of the plant.

With citrus fruits, we are especially concerned with chemical sprays, as the outer fruit skin is squeezed to produce the oils, collecting a high concentration of chemical spray in the oil. This is why it is so important to use only organic oils. We must avoid introducing any chemical toxins into the body along with the precious medicine it needs.[1] The Oath of Hippocrates reminds us that first and foremost, when we try to help someone, we certainly don't want to cause them any harm by introducing poisonous materials into their body.

In organic agriculture, quality methods are employed to obtain a superior looking product, which will be purchased by visual appeal such as attractive fruits or vegetables. In purchasing essential oils however, there is almost no visual dimension. We don't see the plants that were used (unless we visit the plantation), only a liquid, a bottle and a label. Initially, only your nose can actually determine the quality. But in the long run, we can know the quality of essential oils during and after a treatment from more advanced fragrance response and observed effects, and by purchasing them from a well known and highly reliable supplier who provides consistently high quality oils.

When the label says "organic," be aware that this is unfortunately not an absolute guarantee of quality. The organic factor alone does not make an essential oil a high-quality medicine suitable for use in an aromatherapy treatment, or a quality cosmetic ingredient. It is of course of paramount importance that the plants be free of chemicals, but in addition, the other important quality factors regarding the health of the plant and care in harvesting, extraction and storage are absolutely vital in obtaining an essential oil with the therapeutic potency and aromatic qualities we need for effective healing treatment.

Cost Considerations

When looking at the cost of various essential oils, it is very helpful and far more accurate economically to see this cost strictly on a **per-treatment** basis. One aromatherapy treatment generally requires no more than 10 drops of pure essential oil, and each ml of essential oil contains about 30 drops.

As an example, a 5 ml bottle contains about 150 drops, which is enough essential oil for at least 15 treatments. So, divide the cost of a 5 ml bottle by 15 to determine the cost per treatment. If it is a quality essential oil, this is the cost for a therapeutically powerful and aromatically enjoyable medicine, which will go to work effectively in the body for three days before being eliminated.

Shelf Life and Storage

The shelf life for essential oils that are used professionally is about two years for citrus oils, and three years for most steam distilled varieties. Oils from woods, roots, barks and resins can last much longer. Most Absolutes have very good "tenacity" and enjoy a shelf life of about five years. All of the oils can be used on a personal basis for many years longer, with a varying loss of medicinal quality, aromatic potency and bouquet. Essential oils never actually "go bad," they simply lose their life force over a period of time as the natural components dissipate.

Proper storage techniques include the use of "ultra-violet," cobalt blue or amber glass bottles with a minimum of air inside the bottle and a cool surrounding temperature. Never store your oils in plastic bottles. Refrigeration is usually not necessary unless the air temperature is consistently high. Never leave your precious oils in direct sunlight, or in the trunk or glove compartment of a car, where they may be excessively heated.

Jacob Lorber (Graz, Austria 1800-1864) discovered in his scientific investigations that natural healing substances are not only protected, but also empowered and refined when placed in "deep violet" glass. According to bio-photon scientist Dr. Hugo Noggli (Ependes, Switzerland), the violet spectral range represents the highest energy domain, and permanently activates and energizes the structure of organic molecules. Special "ultra-violet" glass for the manufacture of bottles and jars has been scientifically developed based on this principle. These are the very best containers known for storage and longevity, and they enhance the life force of essential oils, creams and other natural healing products.

Measurable Life-Force Frequencies

Some research has begun which indicates that therapeutic quality essential oils carry a measurable bio-electric frequency. In 1992, Dr. Gary Young of Young Living, and Bruce Tainio of Tainio Technology, began to accurately measure the electrical frequency of various essential oils. Their initial findings contend that all of the oils have a bio-electric frequency measurable in hertz, megahertz and kilohertz. Frequency is a measurable rate of electrical energy that is constant between two points, and every living thing theoretically has a measurable electrical frequency. Tainio invented and built a special machine to make these measurements, called a BT3 Frequency Monitoring System. This device used a highly refined sensor to measure bio-electrical frequencies of plant nutrients and essential oils.

Essential oils apparently contain electrical frequencies that are several times greater than the frequency of herbs or food. Raw foods, for example, have been shown to have a frequency of about 29 hertz (hz), while cooked foods have a frequency ranging from 0 to 15 hz. Dry herbs range from 15 to 22 hz, fresh herbs from 20 to 27 hz. Essential oils start at 50 hz (birch), and go as high as 320 hz (rose otto). Rose oil has the highest frequency, and also the greatest spiritual power of all fragrances, according to Shoshanna Harrari, a master healer based in Israel. Young and Tainio discovered that a healthy body from head to foot has a frequency ranging from 62 to 71 hz. The abdomen resonates at 59 to 62 hz. The area from the sternum to the upper throat resonates at about 62 to 68 hz, while the head area of a normal healthy person resonates at 72 to 78 hz. This head area measurement can range as high as 90 hz during times of extreme mental activity. These measurements were recorded by use of the BT3 Frequency Monitoring System.

Disease begins at 58 hz, and becomes more severe at lower measurements. Cancer has a frequency of 42 hz. A radiologist from Sweden discovered in the 1980s that by putting an electrode inside a tumor and running a direct current through it, he could dissolve the cancer tumor and stop its growth.[2] Initial findings support the theory that headaches are caused by a disturbance in the electrical fields between the right and left lobes of the brain, when the frequency between the two lobes varies by more than 3 hz. If the frequency varies by more than 10 hz, substantial migraine headaches can occur. In the early 1920s, Royal Raymond Rife MD developed a "frequency generator." According to Dr. Rife, every disease has a specific frequency. It was discovered that a living substance with a higher frequency would destroy any disease, which would always have a frequency of 58 hz or less.[3] Royal Rife's work was very controversial in his time, and his notes, records and machinery were apparently either confiscated or destroyed.

Energetic and vibrational aromatherapy involves setting up just the right environment for the treatment, and can include music, sounds, color and of course fragrances.[4] Clinical research shows that essential oils have some of the highest frequencies of all natural organic substances. Introducing the oils to the body in various ways, especially in several consistent applications, helps to create and maintain an optimal frequency and environment in which disease, bacteria, virus and fungus cannot exist. This is all assuming that the essential oils are natural, fresh, of the highest quality, and free of impurities – these oils will have (or will be able to maintain) a consistently high frequency, and be the most useful for healing.[5]

Chapter 8

Fragrance Testing: The Key to Aromatherapy

Have you ever been asked to be a matchmaker? If a good friend who needs your help wanted to "meet someone," in order to assist them you would want to think carefully about all of your other friends, hoping to zero in on someone who might be just the right choice. When the two finally meet for a date, it is usually clear almost immediately whether or not there is good "chemistry" between them. This matchmaking process is remarkably similar to the art of choosing the correct essential oils for a friend, a client, or for yourself. In selecting essential oils, think of the oil as a "person" you would like to introduce as a potentially good match. Every essential oil actually has a unique "personality" and "soul." As we get to know each one in our collection, we become more personally acquainted with the unique inner nature and character of each fragrance.

When we first experience the essential oil, this is like a first date. The chemistry between the oil and the client will usually become clear immediately, according to the way they respond to the fragrance. This is only a brief encounter compared to using the essential oil in an aromatherapy treatment, but it is a very reliable first impression. If the client is drawn to the fragrance, it will be effective and enjoyable when they use it in a treatment right at that time. If they are not drawn to it, the oil should not be used at that time, but might still be an appropriate choice when used in a later treatment, *if* it tests positively later.

It is important to realize that our preferences (and needs) for the oils are continuously changing. We will be attracted to different oils at night than we would choose in the morning, and different oils at various seasons in the year. A woman will be drawn to varying oils at different times during her monthly cycle. As our state of health changes, our fragrance preferences and needs change accordingly. The most classic exception to this principle is our attraction to the Temple incense blend, the fragrance of Paradise, which entices the soul of every person at any time.

Our goal in this aspect of becoming a seasoned and proficient aromatherapist is to learn to become a consistently good matchmaker. When doing this process for an essential oil treatment, we actually try to choose *up to five* good candidates for a *potentially* good match, and hopefully one *or more* of them will turn out just right. We usually try to limit selections to five candidates at most, to not overwhelm the nose of the person who will do the testing and receive the treatment.

Any aromatherapy book or training course can tell us which essential oils to use to treat various health conditions. Yet, this information can often be misleading, unreliable and sometimes even dangerous, without proper matching. It is like a general survey of many people who respond to a given fragrance in a particular way on the "bell curve," but this approach is not reliable enough *in itself* to direct us to precisely the correct oils and formulation to use in a professional treatment. Many essential oils are multi-purpose and can not be neatly categorized, while every person has a unique body chemistry. Also, most physical ailments involve a psychological factor which may or may not be the actual *cause* of the ailment. We often can not readily know from theoretical information alone which oil(s) will help a client the most, even when all aspects of their health condition have been diagnosed correctly.

We need a far more accurate way to know exactly which oil(s) to use, and to pinpoint the precise formulation. A special fragrance test can reveal this information very accurately, because our sense of smell is such a perceptive, intuitive and reliable guide. I have developed such a test over the years through my own treatment experience and observations, and as a direct result of my studies in mystical aromatics. I progressively learned the importance of fully trusting the sense of smell within each person, since we learn that our sense of smell is potentially as accurate and reliable today as it was from the beginning of Creation (as outlined in chapter 1). I consider the fragrance testing approach to be the hidden mystical key to Aromatherapy. I have never seen it outlined in any aromatherapy book, and I rarely meet practitioners who employ this method, or who are fully aware of it, even among those who were professionally trained in aromatherapy.

The key is that after safety screening, the person who will receive the aromatherapy treatment must smell each "candidate" essential oil that potentially *might be* used, to check exactly how they respond to the fragrance. *The more they are drawn to the fragrance, the more helpful it will be in any type of treatment.* Conversely, oils which are not appealing aromatically should not be used at that time.

First, good candidates must be selected by the practitioner, which seem to closely match the health profile of the client. After careful diagnosis, these selections are made based on knowing the characteristics of the oils available, and matching them with the physical, psychological, emotional and spiritual condition of the person being treated. Sometimes, one or more totally intuitive candidate choices can be made. The number of candidates is generally limited to between 4 and 6 essential oil selections at most, to not overwhelm the nose of the client, who must carefully test each one individually. Usually the oils are put onto separate tissues, and offered one by one to the client, **without revealing the identity** of the oils until all fragrance testing is completed.

It is so important to choose the correct essential oil(s) for any type of treatment, and then formulate them properly. The right oil(s) will always be beneficial, but incorrect choices or even the right oils in the wrong proportions could be counter-productive. Before applying essential oils directly to the skin, using them in a massage or bath treatment, or diffusing them into the air, we must know for sure that we have made safe and correct choices. Until we have clearly determined that an essential oil is truly the right match, it is only a candidate or possibility. Never apply candidate oils to the skin in order to smell-test them. Put a drop on a tissue instead. Once any essential oil is on your skin, it will soon enter your bloodstream, and also you may be stuck with an unwanted fragrance for hours.

Making Your List of Candidates

Choosing the correct essential oil(s) and formulation for any type of aromatherapy treatment begins with making a good list of candidate oils. Here is the basic 4-step procedure that I have developed, for making a list of up to five safe and hopefully well-chosen essential oil candidates, and testing them:

1. **Note safety concerns:** Before you start any type of aromatherapy treatment, or even begin to write down your candidate list, the first step is to very carefully study the condition of your client, and take note of any **possible** safety concerns. Jot down **every** possible vulnerability your client might have. Be careful

to never include any contra-indicated (potentially dangerous) oils on your list of candidates. Consult a reliable essential oil safety information chart. One can be found on our website at www.avaroma.com/safety.php

2. **Diagnosis:** Also gather as much information as possible about the state of health of your client by discussion, a visual evaluation, and learn to employ one or more diagnostic techniques such as reflexology, iridology and/or muscle testing.

3. **Choose good candidates:** It is worthwhile to take the time to do this very carefully, as you don't want to miss any important possibilities. Make a list of all essential oils available that might be good candidates for the treatment. Always remember: **do not** initially reveal **any** names of oils to your client, until after testing. A written list and additional notes should be retained for future reference, if you plan to work with this client again. Good candidate oils are best chosen by using a combination of different methods to gather vital information:

   a. **Past experience.** Everyone has some idea of fragrances that they are attracted to, or perhaps ones they have used previously with success. In this case your client will know the name of one or more candidates, but still don't let them know when it is being tested among those being offered as possibilities.

   b. **Through diagnostic matching.** The more you know about the condition of your client on one hand, and the known treatment effects of the essential oils available, the easier it is to make a good match. For this info on the various oils, see listings in excellent aromatherapy books such as those authored by Patricia Davis, Valerie Worwood, Suzanne Fischer-Rizzi, or the organic oils section of our website at www.avaroma.com/po.php

   c. **Intuition.** It is often possible to choose good candidates through intuition, chosen by either the practitioner or the client. This is the mystical approach. I have seen this done successfully many times by passing a hand over the bottles without seeing the names, and making a selection or two. Sometimes a totally intuitive process can lead to the very best candidate for the treatment. But remember, for any oil – until the oil is fragrance tested and approved by the client, it is only a candidate.

d. **Finally, screen all candidates for safety again.** Review the safety concerns noted for this client. Remove from your list any dangerous candidates that are contra-indicated, and which might be a safety concern.

4. Each safe candidate is now fragrance tested by the client. This is accomplished with the following considerations:

a. The oils are tested one at a time, with sufficient intervals. Sometimes it helps to use coffee grinds between oils, to completely clear the nose.

b. Do not initially reveal the identity of any of the oils. Don't show your list of candidates to your client, and don't say the names of the oils as they are offered. We don't want the rational brain involved - the success of this testing method is entirely dependent upon the **limbic brain**. (After all of the testing of the 5 candidates is completed, *then* reveal which oils were tested, and which ones have been selected and rejected.)

c. Oils that get a neutral or a negative response should be put away, eliminated from the list and not used at that time.

d. All candidate oils should be carefully rated for fragrance preference on a 1-to-10 scale. A 10 rating is the most positive response possible. A rating of 7 to 10 is considered a positive response. 4 to 6 is a neutral response; 1 to 3 is a negative response. With any oil rated a 6 or below, don't use it in the treatment.

Finally, the oils that received a positive response (7 to 10 rating) should be re-tested, to optimize accuracy in the fragrance response, and see how these oils compare in fragrance appeal, relative to each other. Continue to assign accurate numerical ratings. This information should be carefully noted as it is crucial in formulating a blend.

For any type of aromatherapy treatment, the formulation of essential oils for the final blend is made according to the relative ratings of the candidate oils that received a positive response. Here are some guidelines and examples for designing the final formula:

a. If only one candidate oil can be found that rates a 7 or higher, then use only that one essential oil in the aromatherapy treatment.

b. If only two candidate oils are found to be rated a 7 or higher, make a blend using those two essential oils. If the oils get an equal numerical rating, use equal parts of each oil. If one oil rates higher than the other, use a greater proportion of that oil in the blend. A massage treatment requires 10 drops total of essential oil, and a bath treatment requires 8 drops total. Let's say for example that chamomile rated a 7, and lavender rated a 9. In this case, blend 3 drops of chamomile and 7 drops of lavender into the vegetable carrier oil for a massage; or, use 2 drops of chamomile and 6 drops of lavender in a bath.

c. If three candidate oils rate a 7 or higher, then make a blend with those 3 oils, again formulating your blend as closely as possible relative to the fragrance preferences of your client. If for example chamomile was rated a 7, lavender a 9, and rose a 10, then for the total of 10 drops needed for a massage, use 1 drop of chamomile, 4 drops of lavender and 5 drops of rose.

The Magic of Synergy and the Power of Blending

One important aspect that gives the Temple incense its special powers is that it is a combination of different spices, harmonizing perfectly together in one blend. Similarly in professional aromatherapy practice, it is well known that two or more essential oils properly blended can be far more powerful and effective in a treatment than any one single oil alone. The essential oils themselves are sometimes called *synergists* as they tend to complement and enhance each other. Like a team of people working together harmoniously, a good blend of two or more essential oils is far superior in optimum therapeutic effect. The potency of the essential oils mixed together is actually much greater than the sum total of the individual oils used, through a mystical process called synergy. This term is derived from two Greek words which mean "working together" (the Greek *syn* = together, and *ergon* = work). Synergy can thus be defined as the *greatly increased effect* of two or more medicinal substances working together harmoniously.

Each essential oil is in itself a delicate and complete symphony of components. This is one reason why fragrances that are reconstructed in the lab from fractions of oils, even when all of the components are from natural sources, are inferior products both medicinally and aromatically. It is vital to preserve the "wholeness" of an essential oil, to protect the natural synergy of all of its components. When these components are altered, the natural therapeutic and aromatic value of the oil is compromised. In addition, even though the original essential oil may have been perfectly safe to use, the component(s) that are removed and isolated may actually become unsafe to use therapeutically, producing side-effects with continued use.

A good aromatherapist can help their client with just one well-chosen essential oil, but is usually looking to take advantage of the synergy principle by preferably identifying *more than one* essential oil that can be used in the treatment. That is why in most cases *five* good candidates are carefully selected and offered for fragrance testing. The goal is to create a blend that will be an excellent match for the physical, mental, emotional and spiritual needs of the client. When the oils are carefully chosen and blended in the correct proportions, as an additional benefit and result, the blend itself will usually be very aromatically appealing, and quite often fragrantly exquisite, especially after application.

A good Synergistic Blend:

a. does not contain any elements which do not belong

b. uses very high quality authentic essential oils

c. is formulated with each oil in the right proportion in the blend

d. has the right overall strength in the vegetable carrier oil (if any)

e. exactly matches the fragrance profile and needs of the client

f. is safe and contains no contra-indicated essential oils

Many people inquire regarding which essential oils should or should not be blended together. While it is true that certain essential oils are said to blend very well together, aromatically speaking, this is actually only a measure of personal preference. To be completely accurate, we can say that *any* essential oils could potentially be blended together.

They all originally came from the same Garden and none of the oils complain or discriminate against each other! They are all at our service, immediately ready to be blended in an endless variety of combinations. Each unique blend should be designed only by the nose of the client, right at the time of the treatment, with the assistance and under the watchful guidance of the practitioner, who is acting empirically on behalf of the client as a messenger, matchmaker and safety guide.

There are basically two branches or approaches to blending. The first, as described in this chapter, is what I would call "medicinal blending," which is the science of making a *one-time pin-point blend* to be used immediately in the healing treatment of a client, or for very special occasions. This medicinal blend can be employed as a perfume, or in a massage, bath, or room inhalation treatment. The other approach is what I would call "artistic blending," which involves the formulation of many types of wonderful perfume, cosmetic and household products, *general blends* to be enjoyed over a longer period of time. These types of blends might be specially designed for use by just one person, or they could be "mass-marketed" to many people who could benefit from them.

The world's greatest "pinpoint blend" is the divinely revealed Anointing oil, an extremely holy Perfume that was designed for very unique occasions... and the world's most powerful "artistic blend," also designed by the same great Artist, is the Temple incense mixture, the most perfect healing remedy for everyone.

Chapter 9

Essential Oils in Healing Practice

Aromatherapy Massage

Massage with the correct essential oils is actually a part-body or full body Anointment. One of the most ancient forms of intuitive therapy for human imbalances, massage is also the *most effective form of treatment in Aromatherapy practice.*

Mental stress and anxiety can lead to a variety of physical ailments, but conversely we can greatly ease the mind by working on the body. When we feel mentally tense, we usually tighten certain groups of muscles unnecessarily. It is important to release this physical tension before the muscles knot or go into spasm, generating even greater mental stress. Massage can easily help to break this vicious cycle. The release of physical tension can soothe the mind, and often lead to a release of emotions as well, especially when we work with essential oils for the anointment that have calming, soothing or uplifting effects on the body and mind.

The use of high quality essential oils in massage treatment is of vital importance, especially when compared to the common practice of using pre-mixed massage oils or plain vegetable oil. When we choose good candidates which are strongly affirmed in fragrance testing, the essential oils will work effectively on the physical, mental, emotional and spiritual levels simultaneously. Adding the correct high quality essential oils to the vegetable carrier oil can make a massage treatment *many times more effective*, compared to using plain (or improperly fragranced) vegetable oil. You will see major healing results that would not be evident at all without the use of quality essential oils.

Mental states may often express themselves in some form of physical ailment. We should consider that there is likely to be at least *some* psychosomatic element in most imbalanced physical conditions. There is much evidence to suggest that people catch colds when their morale is low, and at such times when our defenses are down, we may also be susceptible to many other ailments and injuries.

The great psychologist Carl Jung has written about the "symbolism of illness," the way in which the *form* that a physical illness takes can give us an important hint about the mental state that is producing it. He cites cases of nausea with no physiological cause, where the patient seems to be inwardly saying, "I am sick to my stomach of this situation." In another example given, unexplained back or leg pains and even temporary paralyses may be a way of the body saying, "I can't stand this situation any more." These examples may seem simplistic, but they are drawn from real life cases, and these types of mind-body statements are actually quite common. Once a decision to resolve the mental state is taken and acted upon, the physical problem often begins to disappear. Thus we should always consider a person's mental state before we decide on the candidate oils for a treatment.

Different aromatherapists use quite different systems of massage, depending on their background training and personal preference. Almost all include in their practice two basic movements: the effleurage of Swedish massage, and the deep thumb pressure of Shiatsu and neuromuscular massage. Usually the aromatherapy treatment approach is an intuitive combination of these methods. What is most important is that the therapist has been thoroughly trained in his or her chosen system, and uses it to treat a client consciously and compassionately. It is vital that the therapist takes into consideration the *whole person* - body, mind and spirit. Do not attempt to give a massage treatment if you are feeling angry, tired or nervous, as this can easily interfere and thereby reduce the effectiveness of the healing process, and even cause considerable disharmony in your client.

Human contact inherent in an aromatherapy massage treatment is of the very greatest importance. Essential oils can be very effective in a bath or inhalation, but the relationship between the giver and receiver in a massage treatment takes the potential for healing to a much deeper level. Physical contact is a very potent form of communication. By means of touch, we can convey love, warmth, reassurance, and concern for those we wish to help. We thus enable the client to reach a state where healing readily takes place on all levels.

Combined with human contact, both physical and spiritual, the use of high quality, preferably organic essential oils in the treatment immeasurably deepens the effect of the massage. The subtle influence of the plant essences can help to influence the "whole person" on many levels simultaneously. In this way, we can help to not only resolve immediate problems, but also assist people towards a more complete integration of body, mind and spirit, and this is truly what aromatherapy healing is all about.

It is important to remember that whatever essential oil or blend is chosen, the anointment will also have at least a subtle effect on the person *giving* the massage. It is always important to also take the practitioner into consideration, and not choose any oils which might have an adverse or unwanted effect. Throughout the treatment, you will be inhaling the aroma of the oil(s) you are working with, aromatically creating a feeling of harmony between practitioner and client. The related safety concerns, and to some extent fragrance preferences, also need to be taken into account as they relate to you as the practitioner, as well as the client.

It can be very helpful to the treatment to enhance the environment of the massage. You may want to use an "aromatic lantern" or "diffuser" in the room. These devices will be discussed in detail in the inhalations section of this chapter. The soft illumination of the lantern with perhaps an additional candle may be preferable to bright light. Subliminal relaxation tapes or soothing music may also add a nice effect. As a final touch, a massage of the scalp - if the client is willing - can be the crowning glory to an extremely relaxing or invigorating treatment.

Carrier Oils for Massage

Essential oils are never used undiluted in massage treatment because they are so concentrated; a vegetable oil carrier must always be employed. The ideal carrier should have little or no scent of its own. Trained aromatherapists frequently use grapeseed or sweet almond, and occasionally sunflower or safflower oil. Every vegetable oil has its own special properties. You may want to experiment and blend several varieties together.

Grapeseed oil is light, clear and has no scent. It is an excellent carrier for massage.

Almond oil has a very good emollient effect, and is nourishing for the skin.

Apricot kernel and Peach kernel oils are well-suited for the face, as they are extremely light, absorb well and they are very nourishing for the skin.

Avocado oil and Jojoba oil (actually a liquid wax) are excellent for very dry or mature skin. Use either only at low concentration (5-10% proportion as part of your carrier), about 20-40 drops in 15 ml of sweet almond or grapeseed oil for full body massage.

Olive oil is excellent for muscular and deep-joint problems, and most authorities believe that this oil is the carrier of the original Anointing Oil of Moses.

Sesame seed oil is good for dry skin and the prevention of pregnancy stretch marks.

Sunflower seed oil can be used beneficially in treating arthritis and rheumatism.

Wheat germ oil, rich in vitamin E, is nourishing and excellent for skin care, and is beneficial in reducing scar tissue after an accident or operation. Use only a small amount (10-25% proportion) as part of your carrier oil.

Mineral oil should always be avoided! It blocks the skin pores and inhibits penetration and absorption of the essential oils. Please don't **ever** use it for massage! Most "baby oil" is actually mineral oil, and it is very unhealthy for babies *and* adults. Vaseline (petroleum jelly) should be avoided for the same reason.

Vitamin E oil is very beneficial in treating skin conditions, and in general for helping to promote healthy and beautiful skin. You may want to add 2-4 drops of natural vitamin E oil to your massage oil formula.

In treating skin conditions, use a lotion base carrier instead of a vegetable oil, for treating particular areas. Mix it at the same proportions as a highly concentrated massage oil, depending on the severity of the ailment. A lotion allows you to focus a treatment right on the surface of the skin for a longer time, which is very helpful in treating burns and severe skin ailments (and also add vitamin E).

Mixing Bowl Method

In a short time relative to the shelf life of essential oils, vegetable oils (except jojoba oil) begin to oxidize and go rancid. As a result, after essential oils have been mixed into vegetable oil, they can soon begin to lose their therapeutic potency and fragrance. This accelerated loss of life-force is especially evident with higher quality essential oils. Due to this concern, it is best whenever possible to mix up your massage oils fresh, right at the time of the treatment. In doing so, a massage oil is blended in a very small amount, just enough for the one session. If possible, it should all be used up by the end of the treatment.

Many people who use essential oils in massage treatment use premixed bottles of massage oil. These products when purchased from a market, or blended up at home for long-term use, are not nearly as effective as a fresh blend. The essential oils in the mixture may have lost a great deal of their therapeutic potency and fragrance within a short time, and later the entire product may even become rancid. The person receiving the massage treatment will not fully benefit from the potential healing power that fresh, high-quality essential oils have to offer.[1]

The logical solution, and the most effective way to use essential oils therapeutically for a massage anointment, is to mix only the amount you will need for one treatment in a small mixing bowl. The bowl should be made of glass, glazed ceramic or clay. A small amount of vegetable oil - ranging from 5 ml for a part-body massage, up to 15 ml for a full-body treatment - is first added to the bowl. The amount of vegetable oil will vary according to the area of the body to be treated, but the *same amount of essential oil* is always used: for a healthy adult, **10 drops** total is mixed into the vegetable oil. The mixing bowl approach also allows for a unique, specially designed formula for each treatment. The formulation is always calculated and blended right at the time of the massage, in the presence of the client, and carefully according to their fragrance preferences at that time.

To do effective aromatherapy massage, you will need to acquire a mixing bowl which will comfortably hold about 15 ml (1/2 oz) of solution. Despite its simplicity, the mixing bowl will become one of your most important tools, and should always be used to produce the best "anointing oil" whenever you do a massage treatment. After some experience with the size of your bowl, you will be able to measure "by eye" the correct amount of vegetable oil to add. The amount will vary according to the size of the body surface to be covered. This is an important measurement, because you want to be sure to have enough massage oil to cover the area, yet not so much to cause you to leave any oil behind in the mixing bowl when your treatment is finished.

For a standard full body massage of an average-sized adult, use 15 ml (1/2 oz.) of fresh, high-quality vegetable carrier oil(s). After fragrance testing, measure your carrier oil into the mixing bowl, add 10 drops total of essential oil(s) according to your formulation, and stir well. This gives you a 3% concentration of essential oils in 97% of carrier, a common standard in massage. Use a lower concentration (not more than 1%, or 1 drop per 5 ml of carrier) for babies, young children, or for frail or elderly people. Actually, lower concentrations (3% or less) often give the best results when the problem is emotional.

A higher concentration of 6-9% will be achieved when using only 5 ml to 10 ml of carrier oil, with the same 10 drops of essential oil. The same *amount of medicine* is being used, but at a higher concentration for a more focused treatment. As always the essential oils will enter the bloodstream and circulate throughout the body, but they will have a much stronger healing impact upon the areas of the body where they are directly applied. This stronger blend may produce better results in cases when you will be concentrating the treatment on only one or two specific areas of the body in treating severe physical problems, such as painful muscle and joint conditions. In such a case, be **extra** careful about any possible contra-indications or sensitive skin.

After the massage treatment is complete, the client should have some quiet time to relax. They should be instructed to preferably not take a bath or shower for the next 8 hours, since the benefit and effectiveness of the massage treatment may be greatly reduced as some of the essential oils are washed away. Instead, to reduce oiliness after a massage for those who are concerned about staining their clothing, lightly dry excess massage oil off the body with a fresh towel. The essential oils will then powerfully go to work within the body for the *next three days*, after which they will be naturally eliminated.

Some of the benefits of an Aromatherapy Massage are:

- Essential oils are readily absorbed through the skin.

There is an immediate psychological effect from the presence of the aroma, in addition to the more lasting effect of the oils on the skin surface, and within the body through absorption.

- Massage relaxes tight muscles, improving muscle tone, circulation and lymph flow.
- The flow of "*chi*" or vital energy within the body can be balanced and greatly enhanced in the enchanting anointment experience.
- The direct human contact with the therapist forms a very important part of the treatment.
- Another healing benefit is the degree of inner and outer relaxation experienced during and after a massage. Most often renewed energy and vigor will follow.
- There is an art to *receiving* a massage, just as there is an art to giving one.

Aromatic Bath Treatments

Aromatherapy bath treatments are an excellent supplement to other forms of therapy. This method, after massage, can be the second most effective form of aromatherapy treatment. Water itself has many valuable therapeutic properties, and scented baths can also be an exhilarating anointment experience for mind and body that can be soothing or uplifting, warming, cooling or aphrodisiac. The heat of the water aids absorption of the essential oils through the skin, and some of the oils will be released into the air as an aromatic vapor for inhalation.

An essential oil bath allows you or your client to experience an excellent form of health care at home that can be very beneficial between massage treatments. Some therapists even make bath or hot tub facilities available at their clinic, so that a client can do a treatment or soak as a wonderfully relaxing and warm preparation, just before climbing onto the massage table.

Aromatic baths can give relief from muscular pain and various skin conditions, and act as a treatment for many other physical and emotional imbalances including insomnia, nervous tension, circulatory problems, coughs and colds, headache and even fluid retention or weight loss. In today's world, this form of therapy is also valuable as a means to reduce stress and counteract stress-related illness. Baths can be beneficially combined with almost any other form of treatment *except homeopathy*, as certain essential oil fragrances (such as those related to camphor and mint) can antidote certain homeopathic remedies. A professional homeopath should be consulted to determine which oils would be least likely to interfere with the homeopathic medicine being used.

To do an aromatherapy bath treatment, first check all candidate oils carefully for any possible contra-indications, and complete the fragrance testing process. Fill the tub with comfortably warm to hot water, and add 6 to 8 drops total of the essential oil(s) according to the chosen formulation, just before getting into the bath. Stir for a moment to disperse the oils well. Relax and enjoy! Fifteen to twenty minutes soaking is enough time to allow the oils to take effect and to achieve maximum benefit. Although the essential oils are not completely soluble in water, they are quite sufficiently dispersed in the bath and on the surface by vigorous agitation.

If your skin tends to be dry or sensitive, mix the essential oil(s) into a vegetable oil carrier first, before adding it to the bath. Use 1 or 2 tsp. of a high quality vegetable oil such as avocado, sesame or sweet almond oil. For muscular aches and pains, try peanut oil. Add 6 drops of essential oil(s) to the carrier, mix well, and add just before getting into the bath. Stir to disperse. This method is gentler on sensitive skin, and moisturizing for dry skin, delightfully coating the body with oil. While useful for some skin conditions, vegetable oils are not strictly necessary in most cases, and they can leave an oily ring on your tub which may be hard to clean off afterwards.

Some authorities advise mixing the essential oils into a carrier of dried milk, high proof vodka, or bubble bath mix before adding them to the bath. According to noted author and Master aromatherapist Shirley Price, for underwater birthing the essential oils should be dissolved first in a small amount of powdered milk, adding just enough water to make a thin paste. She also recommends a blend of 3 to 4 drops of essential oil blended into honey or dried milk for aromatic baths of children and the elderly, and using a large bowl for bathing specific areas. The "Sitz bath," as it is known in England, is ideal for treating hemorrhoids and stitches after childbirth. Three or four drops total of essential oil are used, with a hot kettle nearby to add more water as needed, to keep the bath warm.[2]

Victoria Edwards recommends aromatic baths for two, as an intimate way for partners to share a revitalizing, romantic experience together.[3] Along with soft lights and natural aromatic soaps, she suggests that special essential oils be chosen to enhance the simple cleansing routine and greatly heighten the experience. She offers some formulas for a winter Bath, and a romantic blend for that special evening.

Bath Safety Concerns:

Always check for contra-indications, especially regarding pregnant women. Never use an essential oil for a bath treatment if it is contra-indicated.

Sensitive Skin. Certain essential oils may possibly irritate sensitive skin in a bath treatment. People with very sensitive skin should avoid the use these oils, or use them at only half the normal amount (use only 3-4 drops) in a vegetable oil carrier as described above. The number of drops of essential oil(s) can be gradually increased in successive baths, up to 8 drops total, as long as there is no adverse reaction.

Protect your eyes. Once the essential oil(s) have been added to the bath, be very careful to not splash the bath water into your eyes, as essential oils will burn. In any event of essential oil getting into the eyes, apply vegetable oil (*not* water) to a clean tissue, and dab gently.

Never use *undiluted* essential oils in a bath for babies or young children. Always add the essential oils (use only 2-3 drops) to a vegetable oil carrier before stirring the mixture into the bath.

Aromatic Inhalations

Inhalation treatments with essential oils can be used very effectively to remedy mental, emotional as well as physical respiratory conditions. An appreciable amount of inhalation takes place in almost every form of aromatherapy treatment. It is the fastest and easiest way of using essential oils therapeutically, and can also be employed by a client at home as supplementary health care. Air fragrance can also deodorize, combat infection, or act as an insect repellant. Inhalation therapy functions effectively because the oils are highly volatile and easily diffused into the air, and they are readily absorbed by the body through the respiratory system. There are many different methods and tools that can be used to fragrance the air, requiring in most cases a total of 5 to 15 drops of essential oil.

The nose itself is not really the organ of smell - it simply modifies the temperature and humidity of inhaled air, and filters out foreign particles. Our sense of smell is actually based in the olfactory nerve which serves specialized receptor cells. There are two separate groups of about 25 million cells, each occupying a small area at the top of the nostrils. The nasal passages have direct contact with the limbic brain, triggering the effects of fragrances. Our perception of fragrance via the limbic system, where the olfactory bulb is located, has a strong influence on the function of the central nervous system, which in turn affects the mind and emotions. This is why inhalation of the perfect aromatic blend, the Temple incense, was so effective. Mind and emotions can also be greatly influenced by an inhalation of essential oils. For example, anxiety states can be treated with sedative oils, depression with stimulating and uplifting oils, and headache conditions can be eased with relaxing oils.

Essential oils enter the body most quickly and effectively through the nasal passages, so this is the best method of direct delivery to the lungs and sinuses. Deep breathing will increase the quantity of essential oils taken into the body, and ill effects caused by this process are quite rare. In the course of inhaling the oils, some of the molecules travel down the pathway to the lungs and are absorbed by the mucous linings of the respiratory tract, where they can rapidly bring relief to many breathing difficulties. Respiratory conditions such as cough, sore throat, congestion, colds and flu can be most beneficially treated in this manner. Arriving at the point of gaseous exchange in the alveoli, the tiny molecules are transferred to the blood circulating in the lungs, and thus quickly enter the bloodstream.

The basic methods of Aromatherapy Inhalation are:

1. **Inhalation directly from a tissue or Q-tip.** This is a simple method of inhalation, which can be done with 1 to 6 drops of essential oil. This approach is used for fragrance testing, or could be used for immediate (although mild) treatment results. Two or three deep breaths will insure good contact with the respiratory cilia. A few drops on a tissue can be placed inside the pillowcase before sleep to aid insomnia, sinus or lung conditions.

2. **Steam.** This is a concentrated "hot water method" using steam, great for the lungs, sinus and throat. The heat of the water evaporates the oil molecules more quickly, increasing the strength of the vapor. As a result, only about 3 drops of essential oil are needed.

Carefully observe these precautions with Steam Inhalations:

a. Be sure your client's eyes are kept closed, and watch carefully for any adverse reaction such as choking or coughing, caused when too many drops of Oil are used, or too deep a breath is taken.

b. For people who suffer from asthma, use only *one drop* of Essential Oil, because of the powerful effect of the vapor.

c. Always check carefully for contra-indications before practicing this method.

d. Be very careful not to spill the scalding hot water!

e. For safety reasons, it is best to have an assistant.

Directions for the Steam method: To treat respiratory conditions, boil pure or filtered water and add it to a bowl, the larger the better. Wait about 30 seconds before adding the essential oils. Use 3 drops total. If you add the oils too early, they will volatilize too quickly; but if you allow the water to cool down too much, the oils will only volatilize partially. Cover the head with a towel (optional - this helps to direct and concentrate the vapors), shut eyes and inhale deeply through the nose, if possible. This type of inhalation should normally be carried out for a few minutes and can be done two or three times during the day, as it should be for acute conditions such as bad colds or flu. If necessary, re-boil fresh water and repeat.

Clients prone to allergies such as hay fever or asthmatic conditions should only inhale for 30 seconds during the first Treatment; successive inhalation time may be gradually increased as long as there is no adverse reaction.

3. **Full-room diffusion.** This is an ambient, enjoyable and therapeutically effective method which can powerfully influence our mood. This approach can also be very effective when used to influence our mental/emotional state during a massage or other holistic treatment. Here are the tools that can be used to pro-

duce an effective diffusion:

a. **Aromatic Lantern.** This is a simple tool that is very helpful for ambient inhalation treatments. This device is usually made of ceramic, and it holds a candle below a small water bowl. Essential oil drops are placed onto the water. The candle continuously heats the water, maintaining a temperature close to boiling. This allows for a subtle room diffusion of several hours or overnight, ideal in treating emotional conditions, and also useful for respiratory ailments. In addition, this is a delightful way to naturally fragrance and beautifully illuminate your home or work-space. The aromatic lantern is inexpensive and can be purchased from many stores which sell household items. Be sure to get a unit with a large bowl, so the water will not quickly evaporate and thus require frequent refilling. Be sure to keep the water topped up at all times.

   Caution: Be careful that the water doesn't all evaporate! If it does, the Oil(s) can begin to burn and smoke. It is also possible with some models that the water dish will break, creating a fire hazard due to the flammability of the essential oils. **Be extra careful: Never leave a perfume lantern unattended!**

b. **Aromatic Diffuser:** This device uses a process called *nebulization*. It sprays out a fine mist of *unheated* essential oil, and is operated for only about 5 minutes *just before* beginning a treatment. The essential oils then remain suspended in the air for at least an hour or until ventilation. This method offers a much quicker and more concentrated diffusion than the lantern. All of the differently sized molecules of essential oil are dispersed together. The oils are at full therapeutic potency with no qualitative loss (which can be caused by heating), creating a relaxing ambience conducive to the healing process.

c. **Electric Vaporizer.** This is one of the best ways of administering inhalation treatment in a health care setting. This tool liberates the lightest molecules of the essential oil first, releasing the heavier ones progressively. The vaporizer should be thermostatically controlled and kept at a low temperature, preventing the essential oils from overheating, which would greatly reduce both their aromatic bouquet and therapeutic potency.

d. **Spray Bottle.** A quick, easy and portable method for dispersing essential oils into the air is with a simple pump-spray bottle. This item is great for travel, the car or a small room, although not practical to effectively fragrance a large room for an extended period time. The basic proportions of the solution are 90% pure water, 9% pure alcohol (vodka or "Everclear" can be used) and 1% high quality essential oil(s). Mix the alcohol and essential oil together first very well, then slowly add the water (slightly warm if possible) in stages, as you shake well.

4. **Baths** are a very effective method of inhalation treatment.The same is true of a Jacuzzi or hot tub, and the Oils are better dispersed in the water, which is an added therapeutic advantage.

5. **Steam Room and Sauna Inhalations** can be a very enjoyable and effective treatment. Depending on the size of the sauna room, use about 5-10 drops thrown directly onto the rocks. In the steam room use the same amount, placed at the steam outlet. I recommend that you start with less essential oil(s) at first, so the oils will not be too overpowering.

6. **Natural Essential Oil Perfumes** are an inhalation and anointment for the body and soul, and can serve as a very effective and enjoyable mood setter. Perfumes can be an excellent supplement to other related therapy, and allow your client the benefit of using aromatherapy on a daily basis. *It is very important to choose the right perfume to suit one's health needs.* Fragrance appeal and your intuition both play a role in discovering your ideal fragrance. The same Oils that would be good selections for any type of aromatherapy treatment are among the best ones to use in a blend of your favorite natural perfume. We will explore the joys of anointment with natural perfumes in the next and final chapter.

Chapter 10

Practical & Mystical Perfumes

The art of perfumery has always been practiced as a form of healing medicine since ancient times, in every culture throughout the world. All through the ages and until quite recently, the practitioner's approach to the treatment of beauty and health care was completely interwoven. The medical healers in every village were also the perfumers and cosmetologists. True beauty was known to be the experience of perfect health. Most significantly, in the practices of perfumery and medicine, throughout history and until only *about 100 years ago, the materials used were all of natural, primarily botanical origin.*

In today's modern world, things have totally changed. Synthetic chemical fragrances and medications have completely replaced natural products in the marketplace, and the ancient link between anointment and healing has been lost. Most modern doctors are not well educated in herbal medicine, and most cosmetic products available have little or no health care value. In fact, they can often cause health imbalances. Instead of working *with* the body, they most often attempt to paint over and hide any signs of ailment or imbalance.

Most of the perfumes in the market today are manufactured entirely from *aromatic chemicals*, foreign substances concocted from petrochemicals in industrial laboratories, designed to imitate natural essential oils. These synthetic materials have no use in health care, and instead overwhelm the body's own natural essences, creating further imbalance. With their attractive packaging and enticing names, it has become increasingly difficult for the consumer to know whether the many fancy bottles for sale contain medicine or poison.

Ancient History

The word "perfume" is actually derived from the Latin words *per fumum*, meaning *through smoke*. The first types of perfumes which evolved thousands of years ago were in fact devotional offerings of pleasant odors produced by burning incense. We find the concept of perfume closely related to religious ceremonies in virtually all ancient civilizations. High

Priests of the Hebrews and Egyptians could be thought of as some of the first artisan perfumers, as they were trained and entrusted with the right and responsibility to compound richly fragrant substances. The materials and formulations were often a closely guarded secret. The Egyptians associated perfume with immortality, and highly developed the sciences of perfumery and embalming. Fragrances were worn to increase personal power and to ward off negative influences and evil spirits. As a token of dignity, it was customary to place slowly-melting scented cones of perfume on the heads of the guests at banquets. Youths would then shower them with rose water, as liquid perfumes were liberally sprinkled on the head and beard.

Egyptian priests and scholars invented and perfected an early method for extracting plant oils, known as *enfleurage*. They appear to have also discovered the alchemical art of the steam distillation of essential oils. When the Pharaoh's tombs were discovered, formulas for perfumes were found on the walls. The ointment jars and alabaster containers were finally opened after thousands of years, and they still exuded fragrant aromas. There are several unguent jars in the British Museum today which authorities have dated to about 3,500 BCE. Tutankhamen's tomb, which was opened in 1922, contained unguent vases that still held fragrant aromatics.

For many years, Babylonia was the ancient center for fragrances gathered from throughout the world. From India and the Persian Gulf came spices, resins from Arabia, and precious balsams from Judea. Perfumes and fine cosmetics were widely used, principally for the art of seduction. The Queen of Sheba overwhelmed King Solomon with her beauty, enhanced by the seductive quality of her perfumes. Nefertiti and Cleopatra, queens of Egypt, reposed on Rose petal couches. After the conquests of Alexander the Great, Greece was flooded with the fragrances of Egypt and the East. Greek perfume shops were meeting places where politics could be discussed, and with their heightened sense of aesthetics, specially shaped flasks were created by the Greeks for ointments, oils and essences. For the ancient Egyptians and later for the classical Greeks and Romans, the luxury of bathing was often followed by liberal applications of oils and unguents.

Incense was of great importance to the Egyptians, and *Kyphi* was the most legendary. There are many records of the various ingredients used to create this aroma: among these were raisins, myrrh, cinnamon, juniper, cypress grass, honey, wine and cardamom. This incense was used for fumigation purposes, as well as for its aroma, and to alleviate lung and respiratory ailments such as asthma, as well as to treat serpent bites. During the Pharaonic period, scented oils were used for many medicinal treatments: fir resin for burns and celery oil for swollen limbs; herpes was treated with myrrh and coriander oil, and uterine problems with boiled cumin. Relief from headaches came from a combination of myrrh, juniper berries and lotus flowers, applied by massage or taken orally. The ancient Hebrew priests were highly trained by the Egyptians and not enslaved during their long sojourn, and carried precious aromatic materials out of Egypt. They received divine instructions at Mt. Sinai for the precise method of preparation for the holy Anointing Oil and the Temple Incense.

The Modern Shift to Toxic Synthetic Fragrances

Botanical materials continued to be the basis of all perfumery throughout the world for thousands of years. But in a laboratory in France during the late 19th century, the process for making synthetic (chemical imitation) fragrances was discovered, and a whole new approach to perfumery emerged. Scientific and technical "progress" developed new manufacturing methods for perfumes which contained the first synthetic materials, imitating and replacing nature's true but far more expensive essences. Unlike natural essential oils, synthetic fragrances can be very cheaply mass-produced in unlimited quantities. In the early to mid 20th century, thanks to further advances in chemistry, fashion trends, and big business interests, perfumes were transformed from being the product of an artisan practice to an industrial mass-produced cosmetic. Today the market is flooded with synthetic imitations. These rather odd fragrances are in fact totally different substances from natural essential oils, and two entirely different concepts and approaches in perfumery emerge.

The modern day chemical perfume concept is that a person's body scent is unattractive, and needs to be improved by covering it over with what is in effect "aromatic paint." The synthetic perfumes thus impart a smell onto your skin that is very similar to their fragrance in the bottle, which overpowers and covers up your own natural body scent. The imitation fragrance lasts for hours on the same spot of skin to which it was applied, and it will emanate the same smell on every person who wears it. It doesn't combine well with our body chemistry, as it is not a substance of natural origin. These toxic chemicals quickly enter the bloodstream through the skin and respiratory system, where they can endanger our health and even become carcinogenic.

Synthetics in Today's Marketplace

Flowers such as rose, jasmine and neroli give an extremely small yield of precious oil, worth at least its weight in gold. Since most floral oils are so exceedingly expensive to produce, genuine botanical oils for perfumery are relatively rare, and have become hard to find in the retail marketplace. The fancy perfumes sold today in retail outlets, in every price range, are primarily or entirely made from synthetic aromatic chemicals. The manufacturers and marketers greatly prefer these substances because they are inexpensive to produce, the fragrances are perfectly consistent year after year (unlike natural essential oils which vary slightly with nature), and the fragrances last on the body for hours. To optimize sales, the perfume manufacturers hide the synthetic origins of their fragrance materials behind fancy packaging and advertising, and by projecting a romantic and seductive image.

Sacred Botanical Perfumes

Natural perfumery makes use of only botanical plant substances, and this holistic healing approach is ancient and timeless. In choosing a natural perfume, we must carefully consider the therapeutic effects of each essential oil as well as its particular fragrance appeal. We recognize that each of us has been gifted with a unique and potentially beautiful body scent, which will actually have its optimum fragrance when we are in perfect health. We are also blessed with a highly sensitive and accurate olfactory ability which guides us to the botanicals that best support our health and well-being.

Our personal body scent can be accentuated, enhanced, highlighted and harmoniously completed with the proper selection and use of natural botanical fragrances. We know a great deal about the various therapeutic effects of natural essential oils. Remarkably, *the very same botanicals that we would choose as proper therapy for our health care needs are the same ones that will most beautifully enhance our personal body scent.* Natural oils come fully to life when applied to the skin, as they interact with the body chemistry. They reach peak fragrance after 15 to 45 minutes, when they have fully merged with our body scent.

At that moment, the fragrance nearly disappears from the area to which it was applied, while we begin to radiate an aura of fragrance all around us which lasts for many hours. This is the scent of the natural botanicals *combined with* our unique body chemistry. This rare and personal scent bouquet, a blend of body and botanical, is fully evident to others, but experienced by us is a subtle way, with a gentle breeze from time to time of a beautiful wave of fragrance. The same essential oil perfume will create a new and unique signature fragrance with each person who wears it. Ideally it is best to have your own personal formulation, or a very carefully chosen product. This is the ancient holistic approach to perfumery, and it is also a very enjoyable and effective form of Aromatherapy treatment.

Perfume Parties

When I started out as an aromatherapy blender in 1983, my first product line was called the "24 Aromatherapy Perfumes." I wanted to present lovely high-quality essential oils and absolutes as single fragrances and combinations, which would be beautiful to wear, have great therapeutic effects, and offer a natural alternative to the chemical perfumes and fragrances on the market. In those days there were no natural perfumes available, and only one or two product lines could be found in the health food stores that included any natural essential oils. I was fooled at first by a famous enticing line of synthetics that were presented as naturals. Finally I located some very nice quality natural oils that seemed pleasant to wear on the body: citrus oils such as bergamot and tangerine; resins such as frankincense, labdanum and myrrh; woody oils such as sandalwood and vetiver as base notes; and floral oils such as lavender, rose, jasmine, neroli and ylang ylang.

Then I invited a large group of friends over for a perfume party, people who are very creative and love aromatics. We put each of the fragrances on a separate tissue. Then we all got comfortable and everyone gathered two, three or four tissues together (sometimes by design, sometimes randomly) and experienced the fragrance, which made a new, unique blend. Some of these blends were nothing special, some were odd – and some were absolutely heavenly! We wrote down the exact combinations of the blends that we liked the most. Then we passed around our favorite combinations for everyone to enjoy, and requested some name suggestions for each one. We came up with some beautiful blends, some great names to match, and my Aromatherapy Perfumes were born! You might want to try this simple technique yourself, with or without lots of friends, to have fun, experiment with fragrances and invent some new, amazing combinations of your own!

A Few Perfumery Guidelines

Due to the vast multitude of fragrances, perfumers over the years have developed a form of musical notation to describe scents, and simplify the composing of perfume blends. The notes of natural oils have been organized into six major fragrance families: floral, green, citrus, oriental, chypre, and leather/animal. All of these families have smaller divisions within them, and certain ones are combined to achieve the desired effects. A good blend will release its fragrance over a period of time. The first scent to lift from the body is known as the top note; generally, top notes are the floral essences in the blend. The middle note reflects the perfumer's skill at combining spicy, herbal, woody or minty essences with higher floral notes. The base note, also known as the dry out note, is composed of the essential oil fixative that is used to stabilize the blend for the long term – often patchouli, sandalwood, labdanum (floral musk), or vetiver. With a truly great perfume, each of these notes will unfold pleasantly and harmoniously over time, and "lift" exquisitely from the body for a period of several hours.

Blending Your Own Perfume

The mixing process is carried out in suitably sized containers, about twice the size needed to hold the total amount of perfume that you are planning to produce. A colored glass bottle with a poly-cone cap is preferable, but plastic may be used if the blend is transferred to glass immediately after mixing. (Over a longer period of time, a plastic bottle will have a deteriorating effect on your essential oils, and is not suitable for storage.) Create a relaxing, quiet and meditative environment, with adequate light in your work area.

Carefully measure the essential oils first, using an eye dropper or graduated pipette. Gently swirl and mix the oils together in the container, and sample the 100% pure blend with a Q-tip or "fragrance strip." Be sure to keep written notes as you go along detailing the exact amount of essential oil(s) and carrier that you use, to preserve your recipe. Carefully add your carrier (Jojoba oil only – any other vegetable oil will quickly ruin your blend due to oxidation and eventual rancidity!) I do not recommend an alcohol carrier, as alcohol can change the fragrance effect and be very drying to the skin.

At first, add less carrier oil than you think will be needed. Shake the contents thoroughly, and test out your blend. Which component seems to be weak or missing? You can easily shift the fragrance balance at this point by slowly adding more of the missing element. Do this in small steps, retesting each time until the balance you want is achieved.

Then increase the amount of carrier oil gradually, shaking well and retesting each time, until you feel that you have reached the ideal overall strength: not too strong, and not too weak. Final fragrance balancing can be done again at this point, if required. Remember, go slowly! It is easy to add more of any essential oil or carrier, but you can't reduce it, once added - you would need to recalculate the formula and increase the overall amount of your blend.

When your perfume is complete, give your finished potion a glorious final mixing shake. Gently fragrance test it, and if you really enjoy the aroma – **make a blessing and anoint yourself!**

Footnotes

Chapter 1:

Aromatic Elements of Creation

1. *Sefer HaKetoret*, Zohar Amar, Eretz 2002, Tel Aviv, p 166

2.Isaiah 11:3

3. *Sefer HaKetoret*, Zohar Amar, op cit, p 46-50 and teachings of Rabbi Avraham Sutton

4. Genesis 1:26

5. *Bati l'Armoni*, Rabbi Moshe Armoni, Amutat "Nachalat Rachel" 1998, Jerusalem, Vol. on BeMidbar, p 157

6. *ibid*

7. *Pirkei Avot* (Chapters of the Fathers) 4:28

8. *Pirkei d'Rebbi Eliezer*, Chapter 13

9. Genesis 3:1

10. *ibid*

11. Isaiah 25:8

12. *Sefer haGilgulim* 38

13. *Tanya* 26-29

14. teachings of Rabbi Avraham Sutton

15. Pesikta Rabati 23:6

16. teachings of Leah Rivka Sand Soetendorp

17. Rabbi Chaim Vital, *Shaarey Kedusha* 1:1

18. Talmud *Brachot* 43b

19. teachings of Sarah Yehudit Schneider

Chapter 2:
Fragrant Stories of the Bible

1. Tzitzith - A Thread of Light, Rabbi Aryeh Kaplan, Orthodox Union 1984, New York, p 2-3

2. Genesis 3:21

3. *Targum Yonaton* on Genesis 3:21 The other opinions quoted here are those of Rabbi Bachai ben Asher (1263-1340), and Rabbi Avraham Ibn Ezra (1089-1164)

4. Samuel I 28:14, Kings I 19:19, and Kings II 2:8

5. Babylonian Talmud, Avot 5:23

6. Zohar, Volume 1, folio 251a

7. Babylonian Talmud, *Gitin* 57a

8. Gemara B'chorot 57b

9. Rashi, *Bereshit Raba* 65:16

10. teachings of Rabbi Gershon Winkler

11. teachings of Rabbi Sarah Etz Alon

12. Genesis 2-5

13. Rabbi Shlomo Carlebach on Genesis 3:12

14. *Zohar Hadash* 79:4, Book of Ruth

15. Zohar on Genesis, Perush Hasulam 47:2

16. *Sefer HaKetoret*, Zohar Amar, op cit, p 167

17. Genesis 24:63

18. *Zohar Hadash, Noach*

19. *Etz Haim* 18:3

20. Talmud *Brachot* 54a

21. Genesis 6-9

22. Genesis 8:21

23. Isaiah 11:3

24. Exodus 19:6

25. Isaiah 61:6

26. Malachi 2:7

27. Isaiah 42:6

28. Isaiah 60:3

29. Genesis 27

30. *Midrash Raba Bereshit*

31. Genesis 27:27

32. Rashi on *Toldot* 27:27

33. Zohar Hadash on *Shir haShirim*

34. Genesis 37

35. Rabbi Moshe Rosenberg, Congregation Etz Haim

36. Exodus 24:12-17

37. Exodus 30:34-38

38. Gemara *Shabbat* 88b

39. Psalms 68:19

40. Gemara *Shabbat* 88b–89a

41. Numbers 17:12-13

42. Genesis 28:17

43. *Sefer HaKetoret*, Zohar Amar, *op cit*, p 166-167

44. *Targum Yonatan* in *Bereshit*

45. *Sefer Adam v'Hava*

46. *Sefer Hayuvalim*

47. *Perush Yonatan* on the Torah

48. Genesis 4:3-12

49. Deuteronomy 12:10-11

50. Deuteronomy 12:5

51. Exodus 25:8-9

52. *Nefesh HaChaim* 1:4

53. Exodus 25:8

54. from the teachings of Sarah Yehudit Schneider

Chapter 3:
Incense: the Sacred Fragrance of the Temple

1. *Machzor HaMikdash*

2. Exodus 29-30

3. teachings of Rabbi Sarah Etz Alon

4. Numbers 7:12-85

5. Rashi on Numbers 7:14

6. Gemara *Menachot* 50a-b

7. teachings of Rabbi Aryeh Kaplan

8. Talmud *Yoma* 2:4

9. Gemara *Megilla* 14a

10. Genesis *Rabbah* 15:25

11. Proverbs 27:9
12. Exodus 30:8
13. Exodus 30:34-38
14. Talmud *Keritot* 6a
15. Exodus 30:35
16. The Spiritual Significance of the Ketoret, Rabbi Avraham Sutton, Avraham Sutton 2010, Jerusalem, Chapter 12
17. *Sefer HaKetoret*, Zohar Amar, *op cit*, Chapter 5, p 58-75
18. Kings I 10:10
19. Encyclopedia Judaica Vol IV, Keter 1971, Jerusalem, see "Balsam" p 142-143
20. Gemara *Avoda Zara* 3:1, 42c
21. Rabbi Moshe Alshich on *Bereshit* 3:21
22. *Bereshit Rabbah* 20:12
23. Innerspace, Rabbi Aryeh Kaplan, Moznaim 1991, Jerusalem, p 86
24. Talmud *Keritot* 6b
25. BBC News online, Feb. 9, 2010
26. Torah *Vayikra* 24
27. Talmud *Keritot* 6a
28. Gemara *Baba Kamma* 82b
29. teachings of Shoshanna Harrari
30. *Pirkei d'Rabbi Eliezer* 8
31. Gemara *Shekalim* 14a-b
32. Exodus 25:30

33. Torah *Vayikra* 24:5-9

34. Gemara *Yoma* 38a and *Ketuvot* 106a

35. Gemara *Yoma* 38a

36. *ibid*

37. Genesis Rabbah 94:4, Exodus *Rabbah* 33:8

38. Exodus 30:1-10, Rabbi Aryeh Kaplan translation and notations

39. Zohar *Pekudey* 2:222a-b

40. Gemara *Yoma* 54b

41. Midrash *Bereshit Rabbah* 5:8

42. Jerusalem - The Eye of the Universe, Rabbi Aryeh Kaplan, NCSY/UOJC 1984, New York, Chapter 9 note 3, p 110

43. Gemara Megilla 10b and Baba Batra 99a

44. Numbers 7:89

45. Leviticus 16:13

46. Leviticus 2:11

47. Rabbi Shlomo Yitzhaki (Rashi 1040-1105) commentary on Leviticus 2:11

48. Midrash from *Mechilta d'Rashbi* 13:5

49. *Mizahav Umipaz*, Rabbi Pinchas Zevichi, Pinchas Zevichi 2001, Jerusalem, on Gemara *Menachot* 110a, p 6-26

50. Zohar 2:218b

51. *Bati l'Armoni*, Rabbi Moshe Armoni, *op cit*, Volume on BeMidbar, p 162

52. *Mizahav Umipaz*, Rabbi Pinchas Zevichi, op cit, p 21

53. Gemara *Sukkah* 52b, *Micah* 5:4

54. Gemara *Baba Basra* 121b

55. *Shemos Rabbah* 40:4

56. *Tanna d'Bei Eliyahu Rabbah* 5:11

57. Gemara *Eruvin* 43b

58. *Yad Melakhim* 1:3

59. Numbers 17:11-13

60. *Mizahav Umipaz*, Rabbi Pinchas Zevichi, *ibid*

61. *ibid*, note from *Kaf HaChaim*, Rabbi Chaim Pelagie, Chapter 17, note 18

62. *ibid*, note from *Kaf HaChaim*, Rabbi Chaim Pelagie, Chapter 132, note 4

63. Exodus 30:34-36

64. Exodus 30:7-8

65. Gemara *Keritot* 6a-b and *Yoma* 4:5

66. Leviticus 2:11

67. Psalms 3:9

68. Psalms 46:8

69. Psalms 84:13

70. Psalms 20:10

71. Malachi 3:4

72. Zohar *Vayikra* from *Shir HaShirim* 4:16

73. Prayer book of Rabbi Avraham Yitzhak Kook, *Olat Rayah* I, p 292

Chapter 4:
Anointing Oil: the Divine Perfume

1. The Spiritual Significance of the Ketoret, Rabbi Avraham Sutton, *op cit*, Introduction
2. Exodus 30:22-33
3. Exodus 30:30
4. Deuteronomy 20:1-9
5. Rambam, *Mishnah Torah*
6. Exodus 30:32
7. The Living Torah, Rabbi Aryeh Kaplan, Maznaim 1981, New York, p 442
8. Rambam on the Torah, and *Sefer haHinuch*
9. Rambam, Mishnah Torah, *Shoftim Melachim* 1:7-12
10. Gemara *Horayot* 12a
11. Rambam, Mishnah Torah, *Shoftim Melachim* 7:1
12. Deuteronomy 20:3-8
13. Isaiah 61:1
14. Kings I 19:16
15. Kings II 9:1
16. teachings of Rabbi Sarah Etz Alon
17. the *Rambam*, Rabbi Moses ben Maimon, 1135-1204
18. Gemara *Eruvin* 43b
19. *Rambam* on *Mishnah Sanhedrin* 1:3
20. Deuteronomy 30:3-5

21. *Zephaniah* 3:9

22. Malachi 3:23-24

23. Isaiah 11:9, Principles of Maimonides 11-12

24. Isaiah 11:3

25. *Sanhedrin* 93b

26. teachings of Sarah Yehudit Schneider

27. Psalms 150:6

28. *Ben Ish Chai* on *Parsha Vaetchanan*

Chapter 5:

The Recovery of the Lost Ark of the Covenant

1. Gemara *Shekalim* 15a & 16a-b

2. Deuteronomy 28:36-46

3. A Door of Hope, Vendyl Jones, Lightcatcher Books 2005, Springdale AR

4. Gemara *Huriot* 12a

5. Kings II 25:2-5

6. *Emek HaMelech* - Valley of the King, Rabbi Naftali Hertz, Amsterdam 1648

Chapter 6:

Sacred Aromatic Healing

1. Proverbs 27:9

2. Aromatherapy an A-Z, Patricia Davis, Vermilion 2000, London, p 199

3. The Fragrant Heavens, Valerie Worwood, New World Library 1998, Novato CA, Chapter 6

Chapter 7:

Essential Oils: Potent Botanical Medicine

1. Natural Home Health Care, Daniel Penoel MD, Essential Science 1998, Hurricane UT, p 96-99

2. Biologically Closed Electric Circuits, Bjorn Nordenstrom, Almquist & Wisell 1998, Sweden

3. The Body Electric, Robert O. Becker MD, Quill 1985, New York, Part 3

4. The Fragrant Heavens, Valerie Worwood, *op cit*, Chapter 9

5. Subtle Aromatherapy, Patricia Davis, C.W. Daniel Co. 1991, England, Chapter 2

Chapter 9:

Essential Oils in Healing Practice

1. Aromatherapy an A-Z, Patricia Davis, *op cit*, p 71

2. Aromatherapy for Health Professionals, Shirley and Len Price, Churchill Livingstone 1999, London, p. 101

3. The Aromatherapy Companion, Victoria Edwards, Storey 1999, North Adams MA, p 167-8